Introduction

Welcome to Carbs & Cals & Protein & Fat. This unique book has been produced to help you easily see the carbohydrate, calorie, protein and fat values in a wide range of food and drink. Unlike most books in this field, there are a lot of pictures and few words.

The book has many uses depending on your individual needs. Whether you are counting carbohydrate, calories, protein or fat, this book takes out all the hard work. If you are trying to lose weight, it can be used as a quick reference guide to check the calories and fat in the food you are eating. It provides an easy visual reference to over 500 food and drink items.

Following on from the huge success of the book 'Carbs & Cals', which was aimed at people with diabetes, this book includes a larger variety of food and drinks with their corresponding carbohydrate, calorie, protein and fat values. It gives you the ability to see photos of different portions, making calculating the nutrient or calorie content far easier than looking at a list of food and drinks.

We hope you enjoy the book and that it helps to make the process of understanding portion sizes and nutrient values easier.

Healthy Eating

The term 'healthy eating' is widely used, but what does this really mean? Within our diets, we have 5 main food groups. The eatwell plate (on p4) shows how much of what you eat should come from each food group. This includes everything you eat during the day, including snacks.

Therefore, try to eat:
- Plenty of fruit and vegetables.
- Plenty of bread, rice, potatoes, pasta and other starchy foods (choose wholegrain varieties whenever you can).
- Some milk and dairy foods.
- Some meat, fish, eggs, beans and other non-dairy sources of protein.
- Just a small amount of foods and drinks high in fat and/or sugar.

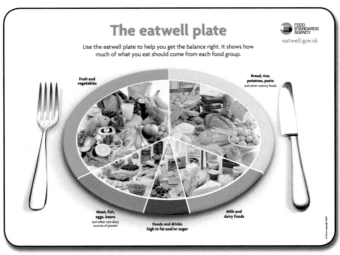

© Crown copyright material is reproduced with the permission of the Controller of HMSO and Queen's Printer for Scotland.

The eatwell plate shows that a healthy balanced diet contains a wide variety of foods from all groups and that some should be eaten in greater amounts than others.

Top Tips for Healthy Eating

1. Eat plenty of fruit and vegetables; you should try to eat at least 5 portions of a variety of fruit and veg every day. 1 portion weighs 80g. As you will see in this book, fruit and vegetables contain few calories and are low in fat. They also contain lots of beneficial vitamins

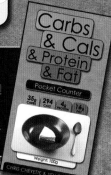
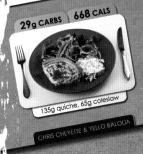
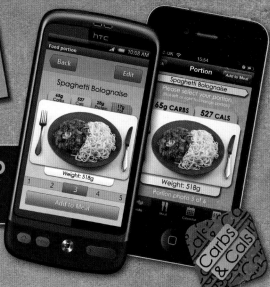

Contents

and minerals. To make it easy to see how many of your 5-a-day fruit and vegetables you are eating, this book includes a yellow border around the portions that count as one of your 5-a-day. It is important to note that you need to eat a variety of fruit and vegetables and that eating 5 portions of the same food only counts as 1 of your 5-a-day.

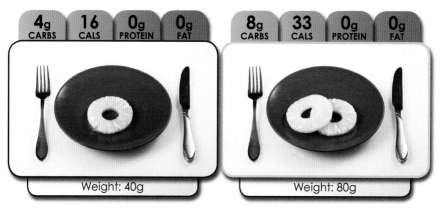

| 4g CARBS | 16 CALS | 0g PROTEIN | 0g FAT |
Weight: 40g

| 8g CARBS | 33 CALS | 0g PROTEIN | 0g FAT |
Weight: 80g

2. Bread, rice, potatoes, pasta and other starchy foods should be included at each meal. Try to go for wholegrain varieties of these foods where possible.

3. Aim for at least 2 portions of fish per week, including a portion of oily fish such as mackerel, salmon or trout.

4. Eat lean / lower fat varieties of meat or fish and limit the amount of processed meats such as burgers and sausages in your diet.

5. Choose lower fat alternatives of milk and dairy foods wherever possible (for example, semi-skimmed instead of whole milk). Foods in this group are an important source of calcium and protein.

6. Food and drinks high in fat and sugar should be eaten in small amounts. They can contain a large amount of

calories and are often the things you need to reduce in order to lose weight and eat more healthily.

7. Alcohol contains a high amount of calories; by cutting down your intake it could help you to control your weight. If you drink alcohol you should spread your intake over the week. It is recommended that men have no more than 21 units and women have no more than 14 units per week.

8. Don't skip breakfast; evidence suggests that eating breakfast each day can help you to control your weight.

Guide to Weight Loss

Before you start to make lifestyle and dietary changes to lose weight, it is important to consider the reasons why you wish to lose weight and that you have realistic expectations about what you hope to achieve. Many people have good intentions but find making changes over the long term very difficult. This is because they set themselves unrealistic weight loss goals from the outset, or they try to make too many changes at once.

Rapid weight loss has been shown to be unsustainable and may even be dangerous to your health. A safe weight loss of 0.5kg – 1kg per week is recommended. If you do not lose weight one week you should not give up. Try to focus on the changes that you are making and remember that lapses are very common.

Do I need to lose weight?

The most common way to assess if you are a healthy weight is to calculate your body mass index (BMI). There are a number of websites which have BMI calculators, or you can work it out yourself using the following equation:

$$\frac{\text{Weight (kg)}}{\text{Height (m) x Height (m)}} = \text{BMI}$$

It is important to note that if you have a large amount of muscle your BMI may be in the unhealthy range, even though you have little body fat.

BMI	Category
Below 18.5	Underweight
18.5 - 25	**Healthy Range**
25 - 30	Overweight
30 - 35	Obese
Over 35	Morbidly Obese

Another way to check whether you are a healthy size is to measure your waist. Your waist measurement should be taken by measuring the circumference of your waist at the midway point between the bottom of your ribs and the top of your hips. The table below shows waist sizes that are at an increased & high risk for men and women.

Waist measurement for:	At increased risk	At high risk
Men	94cm (37 inches)	102cm (40 inches)
Women	80cm (31.5 inches)	88cm (34.5 inches)

If you have a BMI above 25 or a high waist measurement, it means that you are above the healthy weight for your height. This can put you at an increased risk of a number of health conditions such as type 2 diabetes, cardiovascular disease, cancer and stroke.

Studies have shown that losing 5-10% of your body weight can give significant health benefits, including a reduction in blood pressure & cholesterol, reducing pressure on joints and may reduce your risk of diabetes, to name a few.

Calories

Calories are the units used to measure the amount of energy in the food and drink we consume. This energy comes from the nutrients carbohydrate, fat, protein and alcohol. Each of these nutrients contain their own amount of calories (kcal) per gram:

1g Carbohydrate	= 4 kcal
1g Fat	= 9 kcal
1g Protein	= 4 kcal
1g Alcohol	= 7 kcal

As you can see above, fat has the most calories per gram. This is why if you eat a lot of foods that are high in fat you will consume more calories and are likely to gain weight.

People often associate carbohydrate with being 'fattening'. However, it contains less than half as many calories as fat (per gram). It is often the preparation of carbohydrate food (e.g. adding extra fat to a jacket potato, or frying) that increases the calorie content.

How many calories should I eat each day?

The amount of calories a person should eat or drink depends on a number of different factors. These include age, gender, physical activity levels and whether you are trying to lose, maintain or gain weight. It is possible to get a more accurate idea of your calorie needs by speaking to a registered dietitian. The guideline daily amount (GDA) for calories for a female is 2000, and 2500 for men. These figures are based on an average person.

Sometimes GDAs are labelled 'for adults' - these figures are based on the GDA for women to encourage people who need less energy to consume fewer calories.

Why count calories?

If you are trying to lose weight it is useful to have an understanding of the amount of calories in the food and drink you consume. It is also useful to have a realistic expectation of the amount of calories to cut down upon and what weight loss you should expect.

Studies have shown that to lose 0.5kg (1lb) of body weight you need to reduce calories by around 500 per day (3500 per week). This could be by diet alone or by a combination of diet and increased exercise. 500 calories is a large reduction, and it may be more beneficial to look at a 100-200 calorie reduction to start with. By eating a smaller portion, going for a healthier snack or increasing your physical activity it should be more achievable.

If you are currently gaining weight, it indicates that you are consuming more energy than your body requires. This is easily done; for example, if you consume just 100 calories per day more than you need for 1 year, this is equal to 36,500 excess calories. This could mean a weight gain of around 5kg (10lb).

This book makes it easier to see where you may be able to reduce portions or make lower fat and calorie choices to lose weight. The following two pages show examples of daily food intake. Day 1 shows a calorie intake of 2409 calories whereas Day 2 shows a calorie intake of 1715 calories. This has been achieved by choosing smaller portions and lower calorie snacks between meals. This example shows how useful the book can be in helping you realise where changes can be made.

Day 1

BREAKFAST (307 Cals)

Bap (white)
25g CARBS | 122 CALS | 4g PROTEIN | 1g FAT
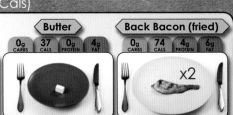
Weight: 48g

Butter
0g CARBS | 37 CALS | 0g PROTEIN | 4g FAT
Weight: 5g (teaspoon)

Back Bacon (fried)
0g CARBS | 74 CALS | 4g PROTEIN | 6g FAT
x2
Weight: 16g

SNACK (201 Cals)

Crisps
20g CARBS | 201 CALS | 2g PROTEIN | 13g FAT
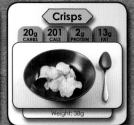
Weight: 38g

LUNCH (644 Cals)

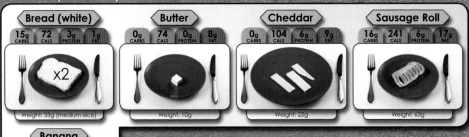

Bread (white)
15g CARBS | 72 CALS | 3g PROTEIN | 1g FAT
x2
Weight: 33g (medium slice)

Butter
0g CARBS | 74 CALS | 0g PROTEIN | 8g FAT
Weight: 10g

Cheddar
0g CARBS | 104 CALS | 6g PROTEIN | 9g FAT
Weight: 25g

Sausage Roll
16g CARBS | 241 CALS | 6g PROTEIN | 17g FAT
Weight: 63g

Banana
20g CARBS | 81 CALS | 1g PROTEIN | 0g FAT
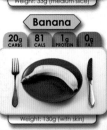
Weight: 130g (with skin)

DINNER (1085 Cals)

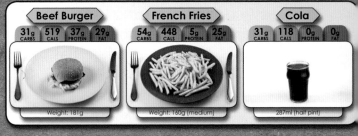

Beef Burger
31g CARBS | 519 CALS | 37g PROTEIN | 29g FAT
Weight: 181g

French Fries
54g CARBS | 448 CALS | 5g PROTEIN | 25g FAT
Weight: 160g (medium)

Cola
31g CARBS | 118 CALS | 0g PROTEIN | 0g FAT
287ml (half pint)

SNACK (172 Cals)

Chocolate (milk)
19g CARBS | 172 CALS | 3g PROTEIN | 10g FAT
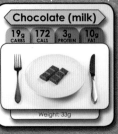
Weight: 33g

including 1 of your 5-a-day fruit & veg

Daily Total
246g CARBS | 2409 CALS | 78g PROTEIN | 130g FAT

Day 2

BREAKFAST (550 Cals)

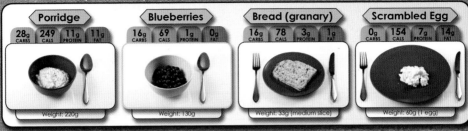

Porridge — 28g CARBS, 249 CALS, 11g PROTEIN, 11g FAT — Weight: 220g

Blueberries — 16g CARBS, 69 CALS, 1g PROTEIN, 0g FAT — Weight: 130g

Bread (granary) — 16g CARBS, 78 CALS, 3g PROTEIN, 1g FAT — Weight: 33g (medium slice)

Scrambled Egg — 0g CARBS, 154 CALS, 7g PROTEIN, 14g FAT — Weight: 60g (1 egg)

SNACK (62 Cals)   ## LUNCH (253 Cals)

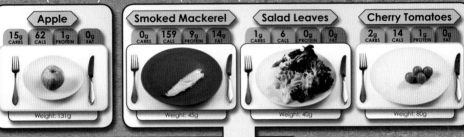

Apple — 15g CARBS, 62 CALS, 1g PROTEIN, 0g FAT — Weight: 131g

Smoked Mackerel — 0g CARBS, 159 CALS, 9g PROTEIN, 14g FAT — Weight: 45g

Salad Leaves — 1g CARBS, 6 CALS, 0g PROTEIN, 0g FAT — Weight: 40g

Cherry Tomatoes — 2g CARBS, 14 CALS, 1g PROTEIN, 0g FAT — Weight: 80g

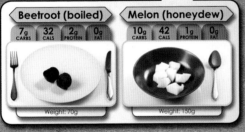

Beetroot (boiled) — 7g CARBS, 32 CALS, 2g PROTEIN, 0g FAT — Weight: 70g

Melon (honeydew) — 10g CARBS, 42 CALS, 1g PROTEIN, 0g FAT — Weight: 150g

SNACK (150 Cals)

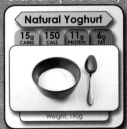

Natural Yoghurt — 15g CARBS, 150 CALS, 11g PROTEIN, 6g FAT — Weight: 190g

DINNER (700 Cals)

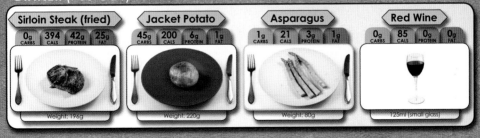

Sirloin Steak (fried) — 0g CARBS, 394 CALS, 42g PROTEIN, 25g FAT — Weight: 196g

Jacket Potato — 45g CARBS, 200 CALS, 6g PROTEIN, 1g FAT — Weight: 220g

Asparagus — 1g CARBS, 21 CALS, 3g PROTEIN, 1g FAT — Weight: 80g

Red Wine — 0g CARBS, 85 CALS, 0g PROTEIN, 0g FAT — 125ml (small glass)

including **5** of your **5-a-day** fruit & veg

Daily Total

156g CARBS   **1715 CALS**   **98g PROTEIN**   **73g FAT**

Carbohydrate

Carbohydrate foods provide the body with its main energy source, which is glucose. They are made up of both sugars and starches. Carbohydrate is broken down by the body into glucose, which then enters the blood. The table below shows the main sources of carbohydrate in the diet:

Food Group	Examples	Role
Starchy Foods	Bread, potato, rice, pasta, noodles, breakfast cereal, pastry, yam, cassava, and grains e.g. couscous	Provides fibre, especially wholegrain varieties. Also an important source of calcium, iron and B vitamins
Fruit & Vegetables	All types of fruit contain carbohydrate in the form of natural fruit sugar (fructose). Vegetables vary in the amount of carbohydrate they contain but are generally slowly absorbed and do not need to be counted	A great source of vitamins, minerals and fibre
Dairy Foods	Milk, yoghurt, and ice cream all contain milk sugar (lactose)	Provides an important source of calcium, vitamins A and B12. Also a source of protein
Sugary Foods & Drinks	Sugar, jam, marmalade, honey, soft drinks, sweets, cakes, biscuits and chocolates	No nutritional benefits other than providing additional calories

For a healthy diet you should have the majority of the carbohydrate you eat come from starchy foods such as cereal, pasta, rice, potatoes and bread. Sugary foods such as fizzy drinks, sweets and sugar give little nutritional benefit apart from giving us energy and should be eaten only occasionally.

It is a common misconception that to lose weight you need to eat a low carbohydrate diet. The food pictures in this book clearly show that the calories in starchy food such as bread or rice are not in themselves high. Indeed foods which are high in fat have a much higher calorie content gram-for-gram:

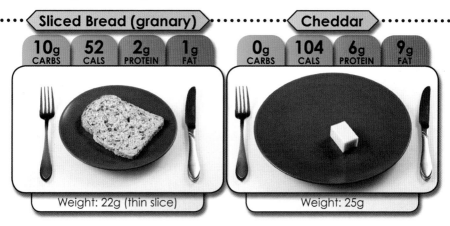

Sliced Bread (granary)				Cheddar			
10g CARBS	52 CALS	2g PROTEIN	1g FAT	0g CARBS	104 CALS	6g PROTEIN	9g FAT

Weight: 22g (thin slice)   Weight: 25g

The way in which carbohydrate foods are cooked or the amount of fat that is added to them is often why carbohydrates can become high in calories (e.g. deep fried chips).

Studies that have looked at very low carbohydrate diets, compared to conventional low fat diets, have found no difference in weight loss between groups at 1 year. The long-term safety of low carbohydrate diets is also in doubt.

How much carbohydrate should I eat each day?

The amount of carbohydrate we should eat in a day varies from person to person depending on your activity levels, gender, age and weight. Around 50% of our energy should come from carbohydrate. The following table shows the amount of carbohydrate per day for different calorie intakes based on it providing 50% of energy.

Calories	Carbohydrate per day (based on 50% of calories)
1500 kcal	190g
2000 kcal	250g
2500 kcal	315g
3000 kcal	375g

Protein

Your body, for a number of important functions, requires protein. It forms the building blocks of hormones and enzymes and is also vital for growth and repair of the body. The Food Standards Agency recommends that 15% of the calories that we consume should come from protein sources. These may be either animal or plant based, or a mixture of the two. For most adults a protein intake of 1g per kg of body weight is sufficient to meet daily requirements. Therefore, if you weigh 70kg an intake of 70g protein is sufficient.

Endurance and strength athletes are likely to require high amounts of protein in their diet; up to 1.7g per kg of body weight per day. The main reasons for this are to act as an additional source of fuel and also to help provide the building blocks for muscle repair and development. A registered sports dietitian can help give further individual advice on requirements based on your own needs.

Eating protein in larger quantities than suggested has not been shown to improve sports performance or increase muscle mass. The body is only able to use a certain amount of protein, and if a greater amount is eaten than you require the body cannot store this. Eating large amounts of protein gives no benefit. Research suggests your body will not be harmed but people with kidney problems should not over-consume protein. Foods that are high in protein include meat, fish, eggs, cheese, milk, pulses, nuts, tofu and soya based products.

Fat

Fat is a vital part of our diet. It provides essential vitamins and is part of all of the cell membranes in our body. Of all the nutrients it gives us the most energy, providing 9 kcal for every gram. Eating too much fat can therefore lead to weight gain and increased cholesterol.

It is recommended that fat should make up no more than 35% of the calories we eat. The table below shows the Guideline Daily Amounts of fat for men and women. These figures are based on an average person. Your individual needs may be higher or lower depending on your calorie requirements.

	Men	Women
Calories	2500	2000
Fat	95g	70g

As well as the total amount of fat you eat in a day it is also important to be aware that not all fat is the same. There are 3 main types of fat in the diet, which are:

- **Saturated fat:** found in fat on meat, butter, coconut oil, ghee, palm oil, and processed foods. It should be kept to a minimum as it can have a damaging effect on your cholesterol by increasing LDL cholesterol.

- **Polyunsaturated fat:** found in sunflower margarines, nuts, vegetable oil and fish oil (omega-3).
- **Monounsaturated fat:** found in olive oil, some nuts, seeds, rapeseed oil and meat.

Foods which are high in fat will contain a large amount of calories. This book makes it easier to see which foods should be eaten in small quantities, or avoided altogether, if you are trying to cut calories or reduce your fat intake. For example, if you were to swap a sausage roll for a bowl of soup you could save 177 calories & 16g fat, or if you swapped some crisps for sultanas you could save 217 calories & 19g fat.

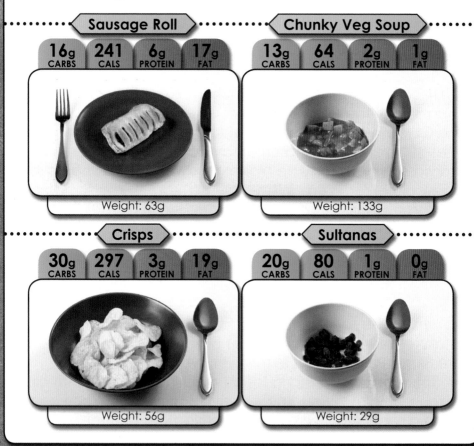

Sausage Roll

16g	241	6g	17g
CARBS	CALS	PROTEIN	FAT

Weight: 63g

Chunky Veg Soup

13g	64	2g	1g
CARBS	CALS	PROTEIN	FAT

Weight: 133g

Crisps

30g	297	3g	19g
CARBS	CALS	PROTEIN	FAT

Weight: 56g

Sultanas

20g	80	1g	0g
CARBS	CALS	PROTEIN	FAT

Weight: 29g

How to use this book

This book has been written with complete practicality in mind. The process of using the book is as follows:

1. Decide what you want to eat or drink, and find the meal, drink or snack in the book.
2. Look at the tabs above the photo for the values that you are interested in. These show the **carbohydrate**, **calories**, **protein** and **fat**.
3. Choose the portion size you wish to aim for (e.g. 150g cooked pasta) and prepare your meal, drink or snack.
4. Add up the carbohydrate, calories, protein or fat values for the different food components to give the totals for your meal.

All foods are displayed on one of the following dishes:

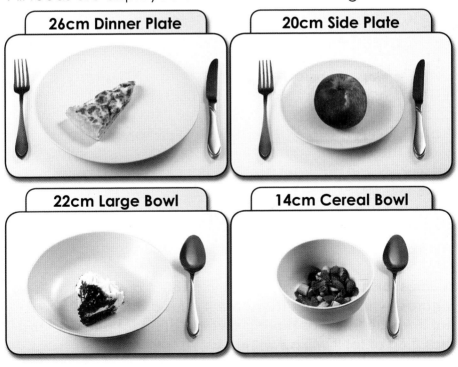

26cm Dinner Plate

20cm Side Plate

22cm Large Bowl

14cm Cereal Bowl

Each picture displays either a knife & fork, or a dessert spoon to help with scale. It may be a good idea to measure your own crockery to see how the size of your plates and bowls compares with the ones in the pictures, and possibly choose plates and bowls of a similar size to the ones shown to make it as easy as possible.

Foods are arranged in alphabetical sections of Biscuits & Crackers; Bread; Breakfast; Cakes & Bakery; Desserts; Drinks; Eggs & Cheese; Fruit; Meals; Meal Accompaniments; Meat, Chicken & Fish; Potatoes; Rice, Pasta & Grains; Sauces & Spreads; Snacks & Confectionery; Take-away Foods; and Vegetables & Pulses. The different sections are coloured so it's easy to find the food or drink you are looking for.

If you are eating a meal with more than one food or drink (e.g. roast dinner, or cooked breakfast), you will need to find each component in the book and add them up separately. For example, your roast dinner may comprise of roast chicken from p177, yorkshire puddings from p168, stuffing from p168, roast potatoes from p200, parsnips from p276, and cranberry sauce from p228.

Each food has 1 to 6 portion examples, so you can easily judge the nutrient values in your particular portion just by looking at the different photos. For example, a digestive biscuit is always the same size, so only 1 photo has been included. However, there are 6 different portion pictures of lasagne included so that you can choose the portion that is closest to the portion on your plate.

Values for carbohydrate, protein and fat are given to the nearest whole gram. Therefore if a food only has 0.4g of fat it will be listed as having a value of 0g fat and if a food has 0.6g of fat it will be written as 1g fat.

The carbohydrate value is always in a green tab, the calorie value is in a blue tab, protein is always in the orange tab and fat is always in the pink tab, so it's easy to see the values you are looking for.

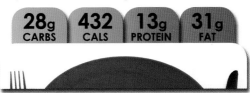

| 28g CARBS | 432 CALS | 13g PROTEIN | 31g FAT |

The weight of each portion is stated below each photo, just in case you want to double-check the weight of your own portion. **This is always the cooked / prepared weight.**

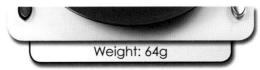

Weight: 64g

For foods that you are likely to have several of, there is a table with the carbs, cals, protein and fat for 1, 2, 3 and 4 pieces, to make it even easier for you to add up.

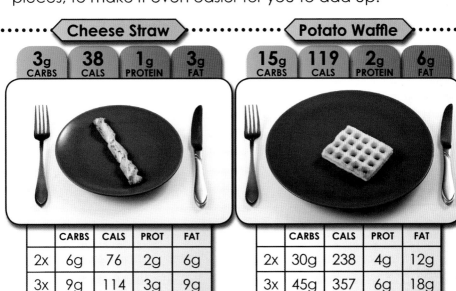

Cheese Straw

| 3g CARBS | 38 CALS | 1g PROTEIN | 3g FAT |

	CARBS	CALS	PROT	FAT
2x	6g	76	2g	6g
3x	9g	114	3g	9g
4x	12g	152	4g	12g
Weight: 7g				

Potato Waffle

| 15g CARBS | 119 CALS | 2g PROTEIN | 6g FAT |

	CARBS	CALS	PROT	FAT
2x	30g	238	4g	12g
3x	45g	357	6g	18g
4x	60g	476	8g	24g
Weight: 49g				

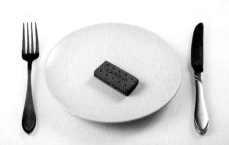

Bourbon Cream

8g CARBS	58 CALS	1g PROTEIN	3g FAT

	CARBS	CALS	PROT	FAT
2x	16g	116	2g	6g
3x	24g	174	3g	9g
4x	32g	232	4g	12g
Weight: 12g				

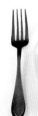
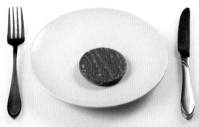

Chocolate Digestive

10g CARBS	74 CALS	1g PROTEIN	4g FAT

	CARBS	CALS	PROT	FAT
2x	20g	148	2g	8g
3x	30g	222	3g	12g
4x	40g	296	4g	16g
Weight: 15g				

Chocolate Chip Cookie

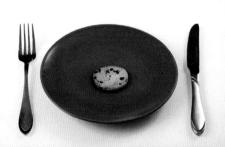

7g CARBS	47 CALS	1g PROTEIN	2g FAT

	CARBS	CALS	PROT	FAT
2x	14g	94	2g	4g
3x	21g	141	3g	6g
4x	28g	188	4g	8g
Weight: 10g				

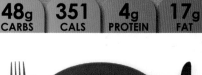
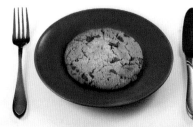

48g CARBS	351 CALS	4g PROTEIN	17g FAT

	CARBS	CALS	PROT	FAT
2x	96g	702	8g	34g
3x	144g	1053	12g	51g
4x	192g	1404	16g	68g
Weight: 74g				

Chocolate Oat Biscuit

12g CARBS	91 CALS	1g PROTEIN	4g FAT

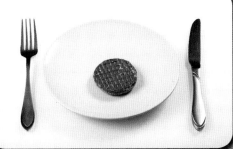

	CARBS	CALS	PROT	FAT
2x	24g	182	2g	8g
3x	36g	273	3g	12g
4x	48g	364	4g	16g
Weight: 19g				

Custard Cream

8g CARBS	61 CALS	1g PROTEIN	3g FAT

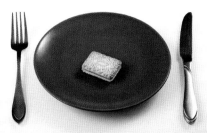

	CARBS	CALS	PROT	FAT
2x	16g	122	2g	6g
3x	24g	183	3g	9g
4x	32g	244	4g	12g
Weight: 12g				

Digestive

10g CARBS	70 CALS	1g PROTEIN	3g FAT

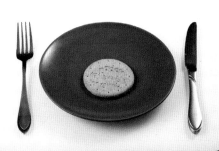

	CARBS	CALS	PROT	FAT
2x	20g	140	2g	6g
3x	30g	210	3g	9g
4x	40g	280	4g	12g
Weight: 15g				

Fig Roll

15g CARBS	79 CALS	1g PROTEIN	2g FAT

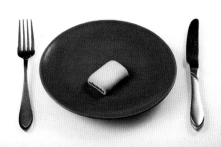

	CARBS	CALS	PROT	FAT
2x	30g	158	2g	4g
3x	45g	237	3g	6g
4x	60g	316	4g	8g
Weight: 21g				

Ginger Biscuit

	CARBS	CALS	PROTEIN	FAT
	8g	44	1g	1g

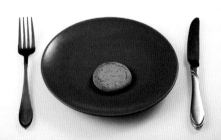

	CARBS	CALS	PROT	FAT
2x	16g	88	2g	2g
3x	24g	132	3g	3g
4x	32g	176	4g	4g
Weight: 10g				

Gingerbread Man

	CARBS	CALS	PROTEIN	FAT
	38g	222	3g	8g

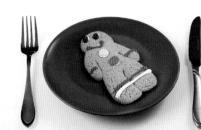

	CARBS	CALS	PROT	FAT
2x	76g	444	6g	16g
3x	114g	666	9g	24g
4x	152g	888	12g	32g
Weight: 58g				

Iced Ring

	CARBS	CALS	PROTEIN	FAT
	5g	28	0g	1g

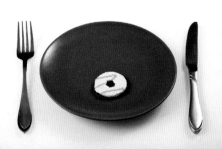

	CARBS	CALS	PROT	FAT
2x	10g	56	0g	2g
3x	15g	84	0g	3g
4x	20g	112	0g	4g
Weight: 6g				

Jaffa Cake

	CARBS	CALS	PROTEIN	FAT
	10g	49	1g	1g

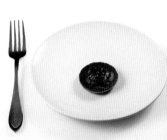

	CARBS	CALS	PROT	FAT
2x	20g	98	2g	2g
3x	30g	147	3g	3g
4x	40g	196	4g	4g
Weight: 13g				

Jam Ring

13g CARBS	79 CALS	1g PROTEIN	3g FAT

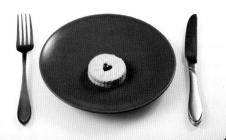

	CARBS	CALS	PROT	FAT
2x	26g	158	2g	6g
3x	39g	237	3g	9g
4x	52g	316	4g	12g
Weight: 18g				

Malted Milk

5g CARBS	39 CALS	1g PROTEIN	2g FAT

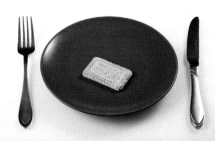

	CARBS	CALS	PROT	FAT
2x	10g	78	2g	4g
3x	15g	117	3g	6g
4x	20g	156	4g	8g
Weight: 8g				

Nice

5g CARBS	39 CALS	1g PROTEIN	2g FAT

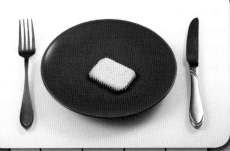

	CARBS	CALS	PROT	FAT
2x	10g	78	2g	4g
3x	15g	117	3g	6g
4x	20g	156	4g	8g
Weight: 8g				

Oat Biscuit

10g CARBS	75 CALS	1g PROTEIN	3g FAT

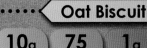
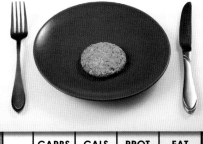

	CARBS	CALS	PROT	FAT
2x	20g	150	2g	6g
3x	30g	225	3g	9g
4x	40g	300	4g	12g
Weight: 16g				

Pink Wafer

6g CARBS	48 CALS	0g PROTEIN	3g FAT

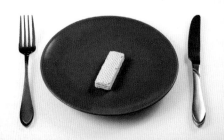

	CARBS	CALS	PROT	FAT
2x	12g	96	0g	6g
3x	18g	144	0g	9g
4x	24g	192	0g	12g
Weight: 9g				

Rich Tea

5g CARBS	32 CALS	1g PROTEIN	1g FAT

	CARBS	CALS	PROT	FAT
2x	10g	64	2g	2g
3x	15g	96	3g	3g
4x	20g	128	4g	4g
Weight: 7g				

Shortbread Finger

10g CARBS	81 CALS	1g PROTEIN	4g FAT

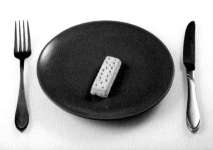

	CARBS	CALS	PROT	FAT
2x	20g	162	2g	8g
3x	30g	243	3g	12g
4x	40g	324	4g	16g
Weight: 16g				

Shortcake

7g CARBS	49 CALS	1g PROTEIN	2g FAT

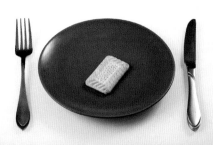

	CARBS	CALS	PROT	FAT
2x	14g	98	2g	4g
3x	21g	147	3g	6g
4x	28g	196	4g	8g
Weight: 10g				

Breadstick

4g CARBS	20 CALS	1g PROTEIN	0g FAT

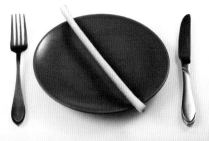

	CARBS	CALS	PROT	FAT
2x	8g	40	2g	0g
3x	12g	60	3g	0g
4x	16g	80	4g	0g
Weight: 5g				

Cheddar

3g CARBS	26 CALS	2g PROTEIN	1g FAT

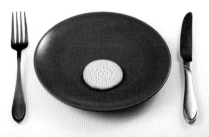

	CARBS	CALS	PROT	FAT
2x	6g	52	4g	2g
3x	9g	78	6g	3g
4x	12g	104	8g	4g
Weight: 5g				

Cheese Straw

3g CARBS	38 CALS	1g PROTEIN	3g FAT

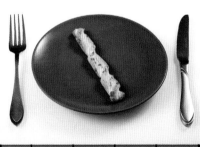

	CARBS	CALS	PROT	FAT
2x	6g	76	2g	6g
3x	9g	114	3g	9g
4x	12g	152	4g	12g
Weight: 7g				

Cream Cracker

5g CARBS	33 CALS	1g PROTEIN	1g FAT

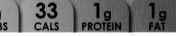
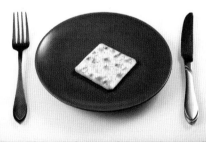

	CARBS	CALS	PROT	FAT
2x	10g	66	2g	2g
3x	15g	99	3g	3g
4x	20g	132	4g	4g
Weight: 8g				

Crispbread

4g CARBS	**18** CALS	**1g** PROTEIN	**0g** FAT

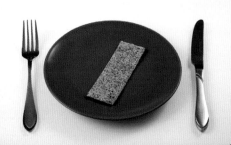

	CARBS	CALS	PROT	FAT
2x	8g	36	2g	0g
3x	12g	54	3g	0g
4x	16g	72	4g	0g
Weight: 6g				

8g CARBS	**35** CALS	**1g** PROTEIN	**0g** FAT

	CARBS	CALS	PROT	FAT
2x	16g	70	2g	0g
3x	24g	105	3g	0g
4x	32g	140	4g	0g
Weight: 11g				

Digestive (savoury)

9g CARBS	**61** CALS	**1g** PROTEIN	**3g** FAT

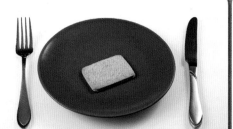

	CARBS	CALS	PROT	FAT
2x	18g	122	2g	6g
3x	27g	183	3g	9g
4x	36g	244	4g	12g
Weight: 13g				

Oatcake

6g CARBS	**41** CALS	**1g** PROTEIN	**2g** FAT

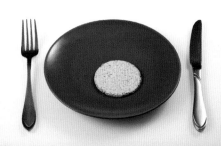

	CARBS	CALS	PROT	FAT
2x	12g	82	2g	4g
3x	18g	123	3g	6g
4x	24g	164	4g	8g
Weight: 10g				

Puffed Cracker

5g CARBS	48 CALS	1g PROTEIN	3g FAT

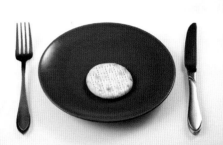

	CARBS	CALS	PROT	FAT
2x	10g	96	2g	6g
3x	15g	144	3g	9g
4x	20g	192	4g	12g

Weight: 9g

Rice Cake

6g CARBS	30 CALS	1g PROTEIN	0g FAT

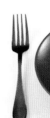

	CARBS	CALS	PROT	FAT
2x	12g	60	2g	0g
3x	18g	90	3g	0g
4x	24g	120	4g	0g

Weight: 8g

Water Biscuit

5g CARBS	26 CALS	1g PROTEIN	1g FAT

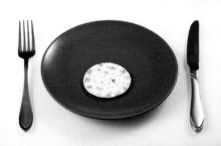

	CARBS	CALS	PROT	FAT
2x	10g	52	2g	2g
3x	15g	78	3g	3g
4x	20g	104	4g	4g

Weight: 6g

Wholegrain Cracker

6g CARBS	33 CALS	1g PROTEIN	1g FAT

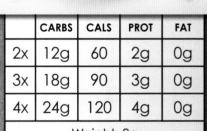
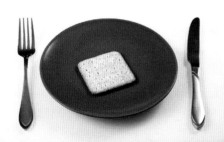

	CARBS	CALS	PROT	FAT
2x	12g	66	2g	2g
3x	18g	99	3g	3g
4x	24g	132	4g	4g

Weight: 8g

Sliced Bread (granary)

| 5g CARBS | 26 CALS | 1g PROTEIN | 0g FAT |

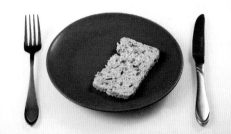

Weight: 11g (thin slice)

| 10g CARBS | 52 CALS | 2g PROTEIN | 1g FAT |

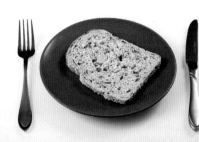

Weight: 22g (thin slice)

| 16g CARBS | 78 CALS | 3g PROTEIN | 1g FAT |

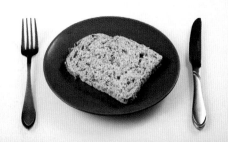

Weight: 33g (medium slice)

| 21g CARBS | 104 CALS | 4g PROTEIN | 1g FAT |

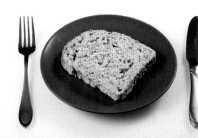

Weight: 44g (thick slice)

| 30g CARBS | 152 CALS | 6g PROTEIN | 1g FAT |

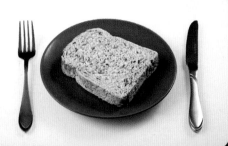

Weight: 64g (extra thick slice)

| 41g CARBS | 204 CALS | 8g PROTEIN | 2g FAT |

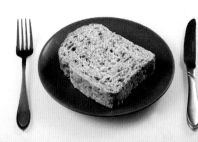

Weight: 86g

Sliced Bread (white)

5g CARBS	24 CALS	1g PROTEIN	0g FAT

Weight: 11g (thin slice)

10g CARBS	48 CALS	2g PROTEIN	0g FAT

Weight: 22g (thin slice)

15g CARBS	72 CALS	3g PROTEIN	1g FAT

Weight: 33g (medium slice)

20g CARBS	94 CALS	3g PROTEIN	1g FAT

Weight: 43g (thick slice)

30g CARBS	140 CALS	5g PROTEIN	1g FAT

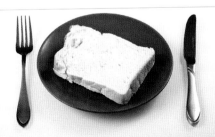

Weight: 64g (extra thick slice)

39g CARBS	186 CALS	7g PROTEIN	1g FAT

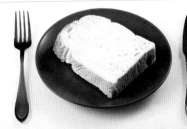

Weight: 85g

Sliced Bread (wholemeal)

5g CARBS	24 CALS	1g PROTEIN	0g FAT

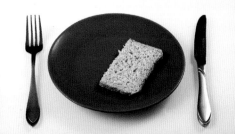

Weight: 11g (thin slice)

10g CARBS	50 CALS	2g PROTEIN	1g FAT

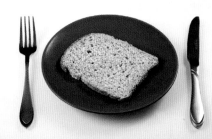

Weight: 23g (thin slice)

15g CARBS	78 CALS	3g PROTEIN	1g FAT

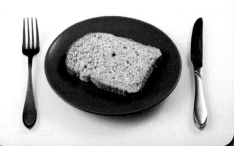

Weight: 36g (medium slice)

21g CARBS	106 CALS	5g PROTEIN	1g FAT

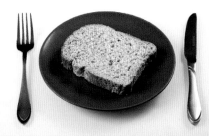

Weight: 49g (thick slice)

30g CARBS	154 CALS	7g PROTEIN	2g FAT

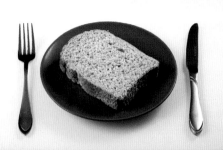

Weight: 71g (extra thick slice)

40g CARBS	206 CALS	9g PROTEIN	2g FAT

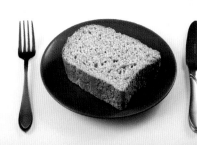

Weight: 95g

Bap (white)

25g CARBS	122 CALS	4g PROTEIN	1g FAT

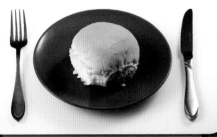

Weight: 48g

60g CARBS	295 CALS	11g PROTEIN	3g FAT

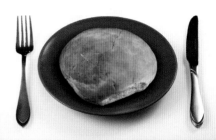

Weight: 116g

Bap (wholemeal)

24g CARBS	124 CALS	5g PROTEIN	2g FAT

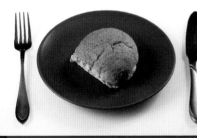

Weight: 51g

53g CARBS	278 CALS	12g PROTEIN	4g FAT

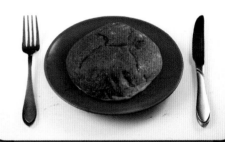

Weight: 114g

Crusty Roll (white)

24g CARBS	113 CALS	4g PROTEIN	1g FAT

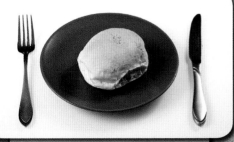

Weight: 43g

47g CARBS	225 CALS	8g PROTEIN	2g FAT

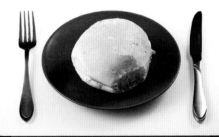

Weight: 86g

Bagel

| 50g CARBS | 235 CALS | 9g PROTEIN | 2g FAT |

Weight: 86g

Burger Bun

| 40g CARBS | 216 CALS | 7g PROTEIN | 4g FAT |

Weight: 82g

Finger Roll

| 21g CARBS | 104 CALS | 4g PROTEIN | 1g FAT |

Weight: 41g

Poppy Seeded Roll

| 26g CARBS | 152 CALS | 6g PROTEIN | 3g FAT |

Weight: 54g

Pitta Bread

| 38g CARBS | 176 CALS | 6g PROTEIN | 1g FAT |

Weight: 69g

| 19g CARBS | 89 CALS | 3g PROTEIN | 0g FAT |

Weight: 35g (mini)

Ciabatta

50g CARBS	263 CALS	10g PROTEIN	4g FAT

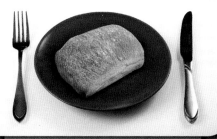

Weight: 97g

Panini

45g CARBS	278 CALS	11g PROTEIN	6g FAT

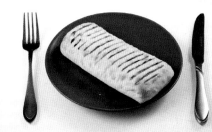

Weight: 100g

French Stick

21g CARBS	97 CALS	3g PROTEIN	1g FAT

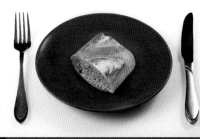

Weight: 37g (slice)

66g CARBS	310 CALS	11g PROTEIN	2g FAT

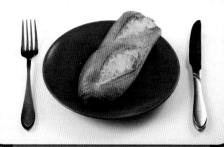

Weight: 118g (small)

Garlic Bread

10g CARBS	80 CALS	2g PROTEIN	4g FAT

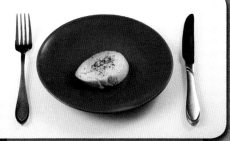

Weight: 22g

30g CARBS	241 CALS	5g PROTEIN	12g FAT

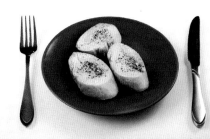

Weight: 66g

Crumpet

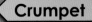

20g CARBS	93 CALS	3g PROTEIN	0g FAT

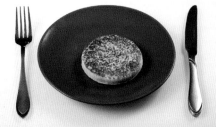

Weight: 45g

26g CARBS	118 CALS	4g PROTEIN	1g FAT

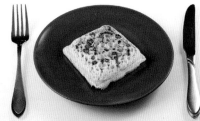

Weight: 57g (square)

English Muffin

35g CARBS	177 CALS	8g PROTEIN	2g FAT

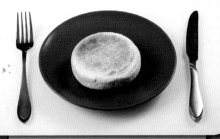

Weight: 68g

Tea Cake

50g CARBS	280 CALS	8g PROTEIN	7g FAT

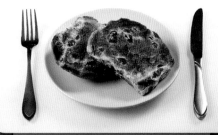

Weight: 85g

Tortilla

35g CARBS	152 CALS	4g PROTEIN	1g FAT

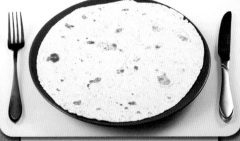

Weight: 58g

Turkish Flatbread

27g CARBS	153 CALS	6g PROTEIN	3g FAT

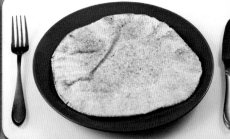

Weight: 60g

Naan Bread

70g CARBS	399 CALS	11g PROTEIN	10g FAT

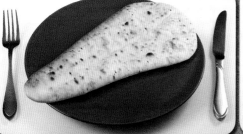

Weight: 140g

30g CARBS	171 CALS	5g PROTEIN	4g FAT

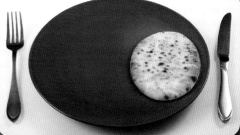

Weight: 60g (mini)

Chapati (without fat)

20g CARBS	91 CALS	3g PROTEIN	0g FAT

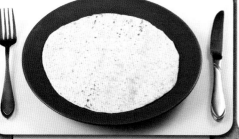

Weight: 45g

Paratha

40g CARBS	297 CALS	7g PROTEIN	13g FAT

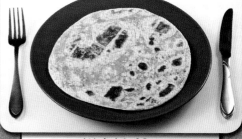

Weight: 92g

Poppadom

4g CARBS	65 CALS	1g PROTEIN	5g FAT

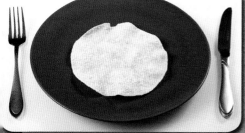

Weight: 13g (small)

7g CARBS	125 CALS	3g PROTEIN	10g FAT

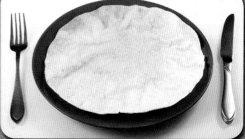

Weight: 25g (large)

Brioche

10g CARBS	64 CALS	2g PROTEIN	2g FAT

Weight: 18g

25g CARBS	159 CALS	4g PROTEIN	5g FAT

Weight: 45g

Croissant

11g CARBS	97 CALS	2g PROTEIN	5g FAT

Weight: 26g

22g CARBS	190 CALS	4g PROTEIN	10g FAT

Weight: 51g

Pain au Chocolat

14g CARBS	142 CALS	3g PROTEIN	8g FAT

Weight: 32g

27g CARBS	267 CALS	5g PROTEIN	15g FAT

Weight: 64g

Toast with Chocolate Spread & Margarine

7g CARBS	57 CALS	1g PROTEIN	3g FAT

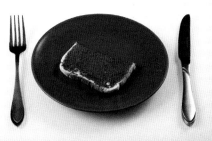

	CARBS	CALS	PROT	FAT
2x	14g	114	2g	6g
3x	21g	171	3g	9g
4x	28g	228	4g	12g

8g toast, 2g choc, 2g marg

13g CARBS	112 CALS	2g PROTEIN	6g FAT

	CARBS	CALS	PROT	FAT
2x	26g	224	4g	12g
3x	39g	336	6g	18g
4x	52g	448	8g	24g

16g toast, 5g choc, 5g marg

18g CARBS	136 CALS	3g PROTEIN	7g FAT

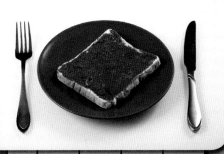

	CARBS	CALS	PROT	FAT
2x	36g	272	6g	14g
3x	54g	408	9g	21g
4x	72g	544	12g	28g

26g toast, 5g choc, 5g marg

23g CARBS	158 CALS	3g PROTEIN	7g FAT

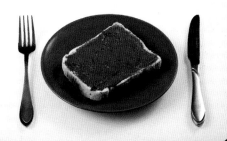

	CARBS	CALS	PROT	FAT
2x	46g	316	6g	14g
3x	69g	474	9g	21g
4x	92g	632	12g	28g

36g toast, 5g choc, 5g marg

Toast with Honey & Margarine

7g CARBS	50 CALS	1g PROTEIN	2g FAT

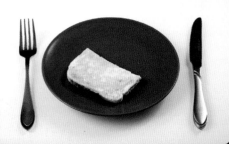

	CARBS	CALS	PROT	FAT
2x	14g	100	2g	4g
3x	21g	150	3g	6g
4x	28g	200	4g	8g

8g toast, 2g honey, 2g marg

14g CARBS	99 CALS	2g PROTEIN	4g FAT

	CARBS	CALS	PROT	FAT
2x	28g	198	4g	8g
3x	42g	297	6g	12g
4x	56g	396	8g	16g

16g toast, 5g honey, 5g marg

19g CARBS	123 CALS	3g PROTEIN	5g FAT

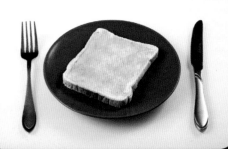

	CARBS	CALS	PROT	FAT
2x	38g	246	6g	10g
3x	57g	369	9g	15g
4x	76g	492	12g	20g

26g toast, 5g honey, 5g marg

24g CARBS	145 CALS	3g PROTEIN	5g FAT

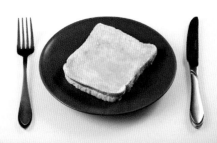

	CARBS	CALS	PROT	FAT
2x	48g	290	6g	10g
3x	72g	435	9g	15g
4x	96g	580	12g	20g

36g toast, 5g honey, 5g marg

Toast with Jam & Margarine

7g CARBS	50 CALS	1g PROTEIN	2g FAT

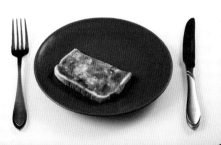

	CARBS	CALS	PROT	FAT
2x	14g	100	2g	4g
3x	21g	150	3g	6g
4x	28g	200	4g	8g

8g toast, 2g jam, 2g marg

13g CARBS	98 CALS	2g PROTEIN	4g FAT

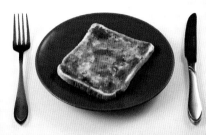

	CARBS	CALS	PROT	FAT
2x	26g	196	4g	8g
3x	39g	294	6g	12g
4x	52g	392	8g	16g

16g toast, 5g jam, 5g marg

18g CARBS	122 CALS	3g PROTEIN	5g FAT

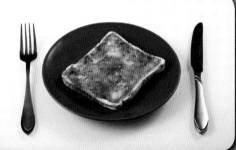

	CARBS	CALS	PROT	FAT
2x	36g	244	6g	10g
3x	54g	366	9g	15g
4x	72g	488	12g	20g

26g toast, 5g jam, 5g marg

23g CARBS	144 CALS	3g PROTEIN	5g FAT

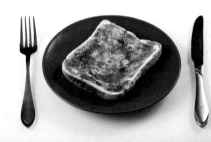

	CARBS	CALS	PROT	FAT
2x	46g	288	6g	10g
3x	69g	432	9g	15g
4x	92g	576	12g	20g

36g toast, 5g jam, 5g marg

Toast with Lemon Curd & Margarine

7g CARBS	**50** CALS	**1g** PROTEIN	**2g** FAT

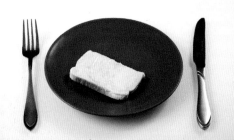

	CARBS	CALS	PROT	FAT
2x	14g	100	2g	4g
3x	21g	150	3g	6g
4x	28g	200	4g	8g
8g toast, 2g curd, 2g marg				

13g CARBS	**99** CALS	**2g** PROTEIN	**4g** FAT

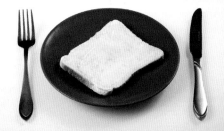

	CARBS	CALS	PROT	FAT
2x	26g	198	4g	8g
3x	39g	297	6g	12g
4x	52g	396	8g	16g
16g toast, 5g curd, 5g marg				

18g CARBS	**123** CALS	**3g** PROTEIN	**5g** FAT

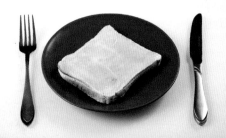

	CARBS	CALS	PROT	FAT
2x	36g	246	6g	10g
3x	54g	369	9g	15g
4x	72g	492	12g	20g
26g toast, 5g curd, 5g marg				

23g CARBS	**145** CALS	**3g** PROTEIN	**5g** FAT

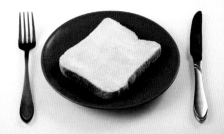

	CARBS	CALS	PROT	FAT
2x	46g	290	6g	10g
3x	69g	435	9g	15g
4x	92g	580	12g	20g
36g toast, 5g curd, 5g marg				

Toast with Marmalade & Margarine

7g CARBS	**50** CALS	**1g** PROTEIN	**2g** FAT

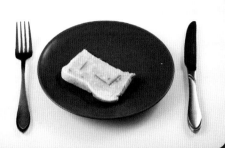

	CARBS	CALS	PROT	FAT
2x	14g	100	2g	4g
3x	21g	150	3g	6g
4x	28g	200	4g	8g

8g toast, 2g marm, 2g marg

13g CARBS	**98** CALS	**2g** PROTEIN	**4g** FAT

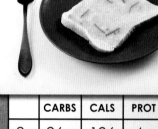

	CARBS	CALS	PROT	FAT
2x	26g	196	4g	8g
3x	39g	294	6g	12g
4x	52g	392	8g	16g

16g toast, 5g marm, 5g marg

18g CARBS	**122** CALS	**3g** PROTEIN	**5g** FAT

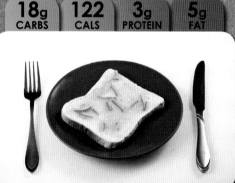

	CARBS	CALS	PROT	FAT
2x	36g	244	6g	10g
3x	54g	366	9g	15g
4x	72g	488	12g	20g

26g toast, 5g marm, 5g marg

23g CARBS	**144** CALS	**3g** PROTEIN	**5g** FAT

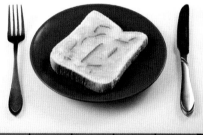

	CARBS	CALS	PROT	FAT
2x	46g	288	6g	10g
3x	69g	432	9g	15g
4x	92g	576	12g	20g

36g toast, 5g marm, 5g marg

Toast with Peanut Butter & Margarine

	CARBS	CALS	PROTEIN	FAT
	5g	58	2g	3g

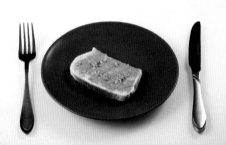

	CARBS	CALS	PROT	FAT
2x	10g	116	4g	6g
3x	15g	174	6g	9g
4x	20g	232	8g	12g

8g toast, 2g peanut, 2g marg

	CARBS	CALS	PROTEIN	FAT
	11g	115	3g	7g

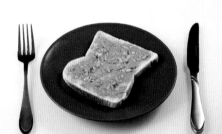

	CARBS	CALS	PROT	FAT
2x	22g	230	6g	14g
3x	33g	345	9g	21g
4x	44g	460	12g	28g

16g toast, 5g peanut, 5g marg

	CARBS	CALS	PROTEIN	FAT
	16g	139	4g	8g

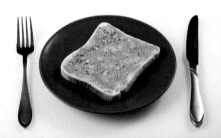

	CARBS	CALS	PROT	FAT
2x	32g	278	8g	16g
3x	48g	417	12g	24g
4x	64g	556	16g	32g

26g toast, 5g peanut, 5g marg

	CARBS	CALS	PROTEIN	FAT
	21g	161	4g	8g

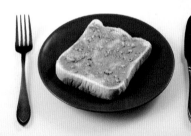

	CARBS	CALS	PROT	FAT
2x	42g	322	8g	16g
3x	63g	483	12g	24g
4x	84g	644	16g	32g

36g toast, 5g peanut, 5g marg

Bran Flakes

11g CARBS	50 CALS	2g PROTEIN	0g FAT

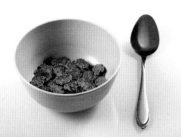

Weight: 15g

21g CARBS	99 CALS	3g PROTEIN	1g FAT

Weight: 30g

32g CARBS	149 CALS	5g PROTEIN	1g FAT

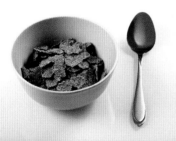

Weight: 45g

43g CARBS	198 CALS	6g PROTEIN	2g FAT

Weight: 60g

53g CARBS	248 CALS	8g PROTEIN	2g FAT

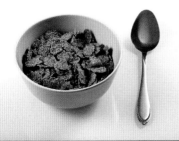

Weight: 75g

65g CARBS	300 CALS	9g PROTEIN	2g FAT

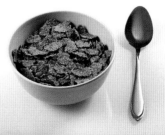

Weight: 91g

Chocolate Snaps

10g CARBS	42 CALS	0g PROTEIN	0g FAT

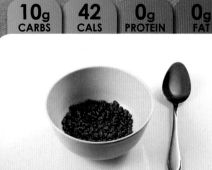

Weight: 11g

19g CARBS	80 CALS	1g PROTEIN	1g FAT

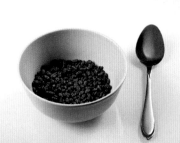

Weight: 21g

29g CARBS	123 CALS	1g PROTEIN	1g FAT

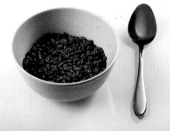

Weight: 32g

38g CARBS	161 CALS	2g PROTEIN	1g FAT

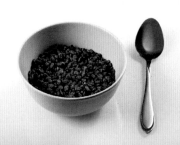

Weight: 42g

48g CARBS	203 CALS	2g PROTEIN	1g FAT

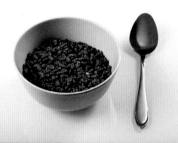

Weight: 53g

59g CARBS	245 CALS	3g PROTEIN	2g FAT

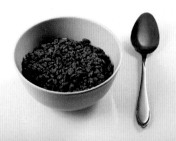

Weight: 64g

Corn Flakes

| **11g** CARBS | **45** CALS | **1g** PROTEIN | **0g** FAT |

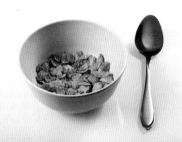

Weight: 12g

| **21g** CARBS | **86** CALS | **2g** PROTEIN | **0g** FAT |

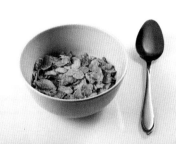

Weight: 23g

| **31g** CARBS | **132** CALS | **3g** PROTEIN | **0g** FAT |

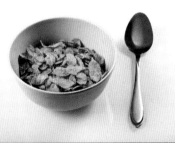

Weight: 35g

| **42g** CARBS | **177** CALS | **4g** PROTEIN | **0g** FAT |

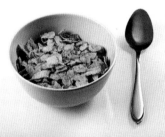

Weight: 47g

| **52g** CARBS | **218** CALS | **5g** PROTEIN | **1g** FAT |

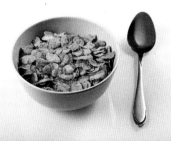

Weight: 58g

| **63g** CARBS | **263** CALS | **6g** PROTEIN | **1g** FAT |

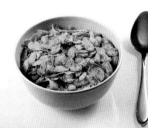

Weight: 70g

Fruit & Fibre

11g CARBS	53 CALS	1g PROTEIN	1g FAT

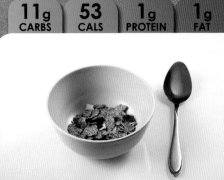

Weight: 15g

21g CARBS	102 CALS	3g PROTEIN	1g FAT

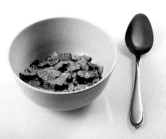

Weight: 29g

32g CARBS	155 CALS	4g PROTEIN	2g FAT

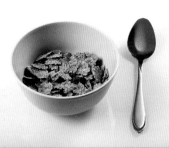

Weight: 44g

43g CARBS	208 CALS	5g PROTEIN	3g FAT

Weight: 59g

53g CARBS	258 CALS	7g PROTEIN	4g FAT

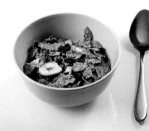

Weight: 73g

64g CARBS	311 CALS	8g PROTEIN	4g FAT

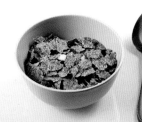

Weight: 88g

Honey Puffed Wheat

11g CARBS	**46** CALS	**1**g PROTEIN	**0**g FAT

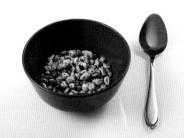

Weight: 12g

21g CARBS	**88** CALS	**1**g PROTEIN	**0**g FAT

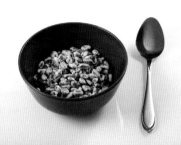

Weight: 23g

32g CARBS	**133** CALS	**2**g PROTEIN	**0**g FAT

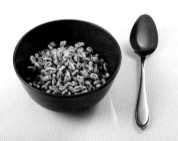

Weight: 35g

44g CARBS	**179** CALS	**3**g PROTEIN	**0**g FAT

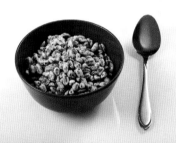

Weight: 47g

54g CARBS	**221** CALS	**4**g PROTEIN	**1**g FAT

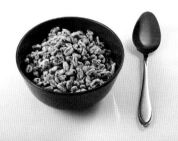

Weight: 58g

65g CARBS	**267** CALS	**4**g PROTEIN	**1**g FAT

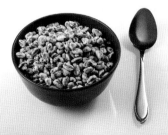

Weight: 70g

Malted Wheats

11g CARBS	**48** CALS	**1g** PROTEIN	**0g** FAT

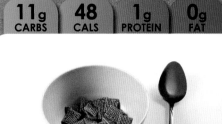

Weight: 14g

22g CARBS	**97** CALS	**3g** PROTEIN	**1g** FAT

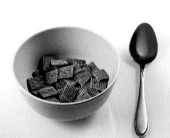

Weight: 28g

32g CARBS	**145** CALS	**4g** PROTEIN	**1g** FAT

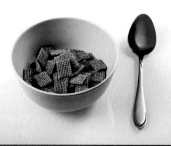

Weight: 42g

43g CARBS	**194** CALS	**5g** PROTEIN	**1g** FAT

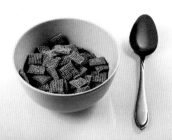

Weight: 56g

54g CARBS	**242** CALS	**7g** PROTEIN	**1g** FAT

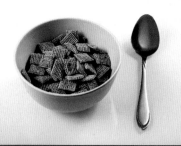

Weight: 70g

65g CARBS	**291** CALS	**8g** PROTEIN	**2g** FAT

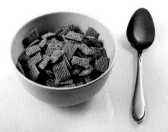

Weight: 84g

Muesli

22g CARBS	**109** CALS	**3g** PROTEIN	**2g** FAT

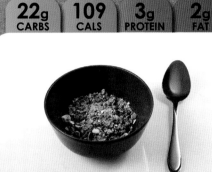

Weight: 30g

43g CARBS	**218** CALS	**6g** PROTEIN	**4g** FAT

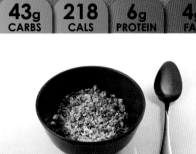

Weight: 60g

65g CARBS	**327** CALS	**9g** PROTEIN	**5g** FAT

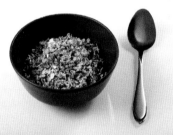

Weight: 90g

86g CARBS	**432** CALS	**12g** PROTEIN	**7g** FAT

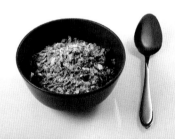

Weight: 119g

108g CARBS	**541** CALS	**15g** PROTEIN	**9g** FAT

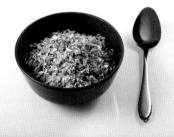

Weight: 149g

129g CARBS	**650** CALS	**18g** PROTEIN	**11g** FAT

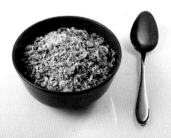

Weight: 179g

Multigrain Hoops

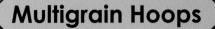

10g CARBS	48 CALS	1g PROTEIN	0g FAT

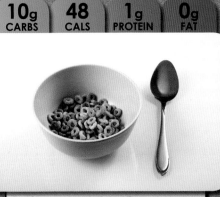

Weight: 13g

16g CARBS	74 CALS	2g PROTEIN	1g FAT

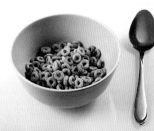

Weight: 20g

22g CARBS	99 CALS	2g PROTEIN	1g FAT

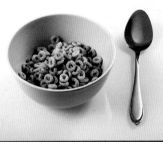

Weight: 27g

27g CARBS	121 CALS	3g PROTEIN	1g FAT

Weight: 33g

32g CARBS	147 CALS	3g PROTEIN	2g FAT

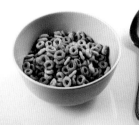

Weight: 40g

38g CARBS	173 CALS	4g PROTEIN	2g FAT

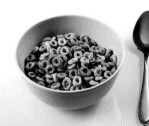

Weight: 47g

Porridge (made with whole milk)

9g CARBS	85 CALS	4g PROTEIN	4g FAT

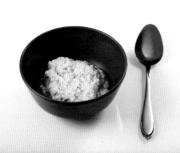

Weight: 75g

18g CARBS	164 CALS	7g PROTEIN	7g FAT

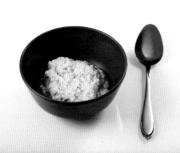

Weight: 145g

28g CARBS	249 CALS	11g PROTEIN	11g FAT

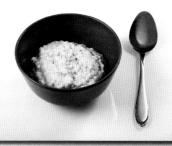

Weight: 220g

37g CARBS	328 CALS	14g PROTEIN	15g FAT

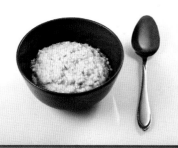

Weight: 290g

46g CARBS	412 CALS	18g PROTEIN	19g FAT

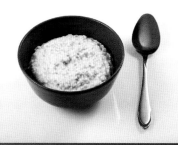

Weight: 365g

55g CARBS	492 CALS	21g PROTEIN	22g FAT

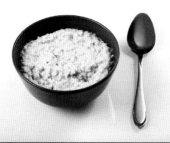

Weight: 435g

Raisin Bites

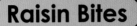

17g CARBS	74 CALS	2g PROTEIN	0g FAT

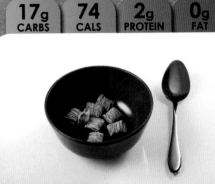

Weight: 22g

33g CARBS	148 CALS	4g PROTEIN	1g FAT

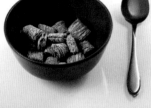

Weight: 44g

49g CARBS	219 CALS	6g PROTEIN	1g FAT

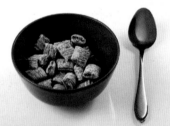

Weight: 65g

66g CARBS	293 CALS	8g PROTEIN	2g FAT

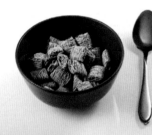

Weight: 87g

81g CARBS	364 CALS	10g PROTEIN	2g FAT

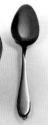

Weight: 108g

98g CARBS	438 CALS	12g PROTEIN	3g FAT

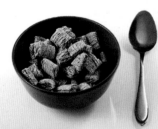

Weight: 130g

Rice Snaps

10g CARBS	42 CALS	1g PROTEIN	0g FAT

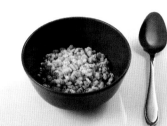

Weight: 11g

21g CARBS	88 CALS	1g PROTEIN	0g FAT

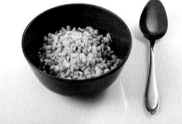

Weight: 23g

32g CARBS	130 CALS	2g PROTEIN	0g FAT

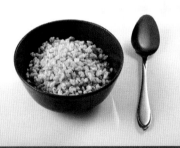

Weight: 34g

43g CARBS	176 CALS	3g PROTEIN	0g FAT

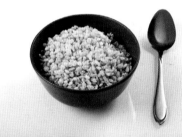

Weight: 46g

53g CARBS	218 CALS	3g PROTEIN	1g FAT

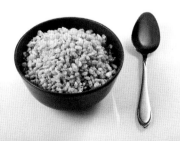

Weight: 57g

64g CARBS	264 CALS	4g PROTEIN	1g FAT

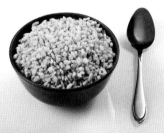

Weight: 69g

Special Flakes with Berries

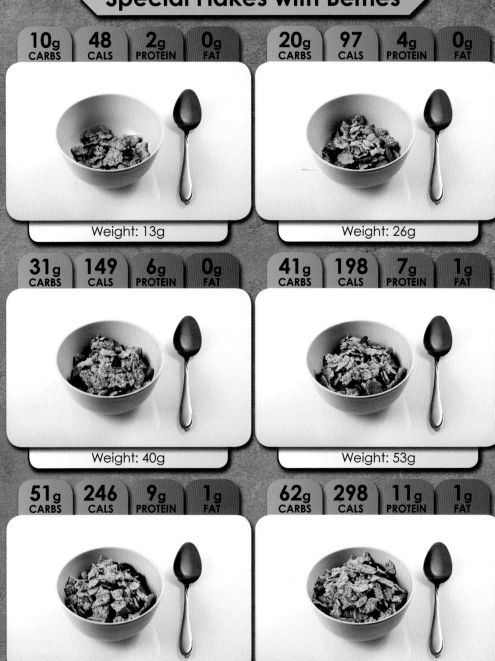

10g CARBS	48 CALS	2g PROTEIN	0g FAT

Weight: 13g

20g CARBS	97 CALS	4g PROTEIN	0g FAT

Weight: 26g

31g CARBS	149 CALS	6g PROTEIN	0g FAT

Weight: 40g

41g CARBS	198 CALS	7g PROTEIN	1g FAT

Weight: 53g

51g CARBS	246 CALS	9g PROTEIN	1g FAT

Weight: 66g

62g CARBS	298 CALS	11g PROTEIN	1g FAT

Weight: 80g

Wheat Biscuit

14g CARBS	67 CALS	2g PROTEIN	1g FAT

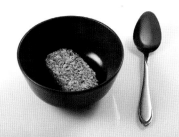

	CARBS	CALS	PROT	FAT
2x	28g	134	4g	2g
3x	42g	201	6g	3g
4x	56g	268	8g	4g
Weight: 19g				

Wheat Pillow

16g CARBS	73 CALS	2g PROTEIN	0g FAT

	CARBS	CALS	PROT	FAT
2x	32g	146	4g	0g
3x	48g	219	6g	0g
4x	64g	292	8g	0g
Weight: 22g				

Oat Biscuit

13g CARBS	75 CALS	3g PROTEIN	2g FAT

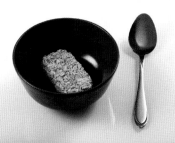

	CARBS	CALS	PROT	FAT
2x	26g	150	6g	4g
3x	39g	225	9g	6g
4x	52g	300	12g	8g
Weight: 20g				

Milk (semi-skimmed)

5g CARBS	46 CALS	3g PROTEIN	2g FAT

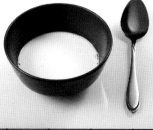

	CARBS	CALS	PROT	FAT
2x	10g	92	6g	4g
3x	15g	138	9g	6g
4x	20g	184	12g	8g
100ml				

Eggy Bread

5g CARBS	97 CALS	4g PROTEIN	7g FAT

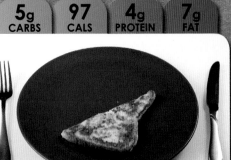

	CARBS	CALS	PROT	FAT
2x	10g	194	8g	14g
3x	15g	291	12g	21g
4x	20g	388	16g	28g
Weight: 25g (thin slice)				

10g CARBS	193 CALS	8g PROTEIN	13g FAT

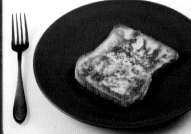

	CARBS	CALS	PROT	FAT
2x	20g	386	16g	26g
3x	30g	579	24g	39g
4x	40g	772	32g	52g
Weight: 50g (thin slice)				

Fried Bread

5g CARBS	80 CALS	1g PROTEIN	6g FAT

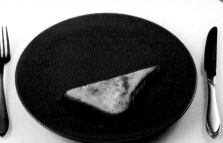
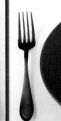

	CARBS	CALS	PROT	FAT
2x	10g	160	2g	12g
3x	15g	240	3g	18g
4x	20g	320	4g	24g
Weight: 15g (thin slice)				

10g CARBS	160 CALS	2g PROTEIN	12g FAT

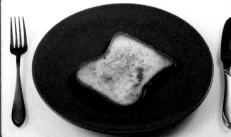

	CARBS	CALS	PROT	FAT
2x	20g	320	4g	24g
3x	30g	480	6g	36g
4x	40g	640	8g	48g
Weight: 30g (thin slice)				

Breakfast Tart

36g CARBS	211 CALS	2g PROTEIN	6g FAT

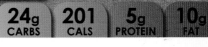

	CARBS	CALS	PROT	FAT
2x	72g	422	4g	12g
3x	108g	633	6g	18g
4x	144g	844	8g	24g
Weight: 52g				

Scotch Pancake

12g CARBS	88 CALS	2g PROTEIN	4g FAT

	CARBS	CALS	PROT	FAT
2x	24g	176	4g	8g
3x	36g	264	6g	12g
4x	48g	352	8g	16g
Weight: 31g				

Waffle (sweet)

15g CARBS	129 CALS	3g PROTEIN	6g FAT

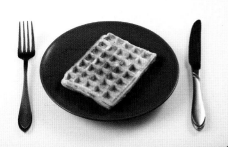

	CARBS	CALS	PROT	FAT
2x	30g	258	6g	12g
3x	45g	387	9g	18g
4x	60g	516	12g	24g
Weight: 38g				

24g CARBS	201 CALS	5g PROTEIN	10g FAT

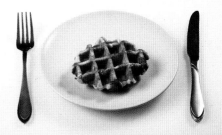

	CARBS	CALS	PROT	FAT
2x	48g	402	10g	20g
3x	72g	603	15g	30g
4x	96g	804	20g	40g
Weight: 59g				

Pancake (plain)

5g CARBS	56 CALS	1g PROTEIN	3g FAT

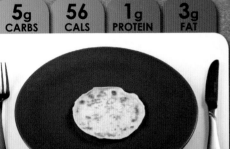

	CARBS	CALS	PROT	FAT
2x	10g	112	2g	6g
3x	15g	168	3g	9g
4x	20g	224	4g	12g
Weight: 22g				

10g CARBS	110 CALS	3g PROTEIN	7g FAT

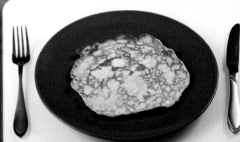

	CARBS	CALS	PROT	FAT
2x	20g	220	6g	14g
3x	30g	330	9g	21g
4x	40g	440	12g	28g
Weight: 43g				

15g CARBS	158 CALS	4g PROTEIN	10g FAT

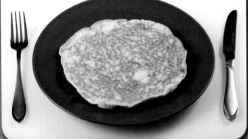

	CARBS	CALS	PROT	FAT
2x	30g	316	8g	20g
3x	45g	474	12g	30g
4x	60g	632	16g	40g
Weight: 62g				

20g CARBS	217 CALS	5g PROTEIN	13g FAT

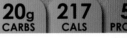
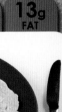

	CARBS	CALS	PROT	FAT
2x	40g	434	10g	26g
3x	60g	651	15g	39g
4x	80g	868	20g	52g
Weight: 85g				

Pancake with Chocolate Spread

14g CARBS	**106** CALS	**1g** PROTEIN	**6g** FAT

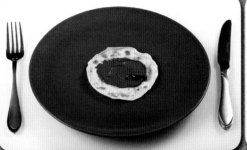

	CARBS	CALS	PROT	FAT
2x	28g	212	2g	12g
3x	42g	318	3g	18g
4x	56g	424	4g	24g

22g pancake, 8g chocolate

22g CARBS	**166** CALS	**3g** PROTEIN	**8g** FAT

	CARBS	CALS	PROT	FAT
2x	44g	332	6g	16g
3x	66g	498	9g	24g
4x	88g	664	12g	32g

43g pancake, 8g chocolate

34g CARBS	**264** CALS	**5g** PROTEIN	**12g** FAT

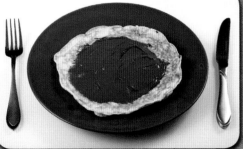

	CARBS	CALS	PROT	FAT
2x	68g	528	10g	24g
3x	102g	792	15g	36g
4x	136g	1056	20g	48g

62g pancake, 16g chocolate

44g CARBS	**329** CALS	**7g** PROTEIN	**15g** FAT

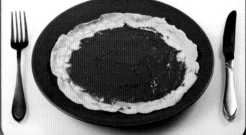

	CARBS	CALS	PROT	FAT
2x	88g	658	14g	30g
3x	132g	987	21g	45g
4x	176g	1316	28g	60g

85g pancake, 16g chocolate

Pancake with Maple Syrup

14g CARBS	83 CALS	1g PROTEIN	3g FAT

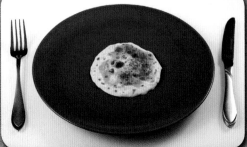

	CARBS	CALS	PROT	FAT
2x	28g	166	2g	6g
3x	42g	249	3g	9g
4x	56g	332	4g	12g

22g pancake, 8g syrup

22g CARBS	143 CALS	3g PROTEIN	5g FAT

	CARBS	CALS	PROT	FAT
2x	44g	286	6g	10g
3x	66g	429	9g	15g
4x	88g	572	12g	20g

43g pancake, 8g syrup

35g CARBS	218 CALS	4g PROTEIN	7g FAT

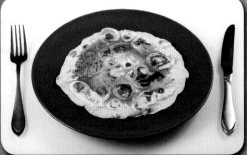

	CARBS	CALS	PROT	FAT
2x	70g	436	8g	14g
3x	105g	654	12g	21g
4x	140g	872	16g	28g

62g pancake, 16g syrup

45g CARBS	283 CALS	6g PROTEIN	10g FAT

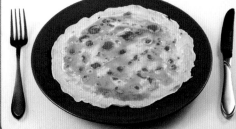

	CARBS	CALS	PROT	FAT
2x	90g	566	12g	20g
3x	135g	849	18g	30g
4x	180g	1132	24g	40g

85g pancake, 16g syrup

Pancake with Sugar & Lemon

14g CARBS	**82** CALS	**1g** PROTEIN	**3g** FAT

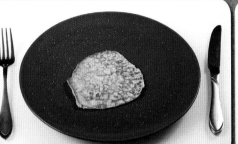

	CARBS	CALS	PROT	FAT
2x	28g	164	2g	6g
3x	42g	246	3g	9g
4x	56g	328	4g	12g

22g pancake, 5g sugar

22g CARBS	**142** CALS	**3g** PROTEIN	**5g** FAT

	CARBS	CALS	PROT	FAT
2x	44g	284	6g	10g
3x	66g	426	9g	15g
4x	88g	568	12g	20g

43g pancake, 5g sugar

35g CARBS	**215** CALS	**4g** PROTEIN	**7g** FAT

	CARBS	CALS	PROT	FAT
2x	70g	430	8g	14g
3x	105g	645	12g	21g
4x	140g	860	16g	28g

62g pancake, 10g sugar

45g CARBS	**280** CALS	**6g** PROTEIN	**10g** FAT

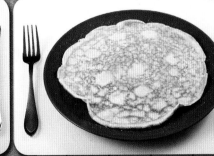

	CARBS	CALS	PROT	FAT
2x	90g	560	12g	20g
3x	135g	840	18g	30g
4x	180g	1120	24g	40g

85g pancake, 10g sugar

Greek Yoghurt

4g CARBS	**113** CALS	**5**g PROTEIN	**9**g FAT

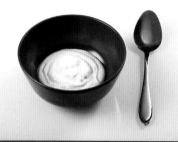

Weight: 85g

Natural Yoghurt

5g CARBS	**55** CALS	**4**g PROTEIN	**2**g FAT

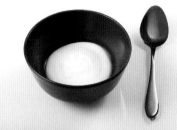

Weight: 70g

8g CARBS	**226** CALS	**10**g PROTEIN	**17**g FAT

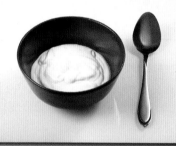

Weight: 170g

15g CARBS	**150** CALS	**11**g PROTEIN	**6**g FAT

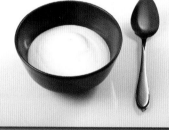

Weight: 190g

12g CARBS	**346** CALS	**15**g PROTEIN	**27**g FAT

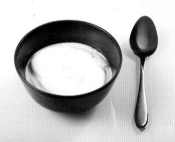

Weight: 260g

25g CARBS	**253** CALS	**18**g PROTEIN	**10**g FAT

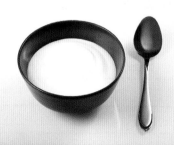

Weight: 320g

Baklava

| 9g CARBS | 79 CALS | 1g PROTEIN | 4g FAT |

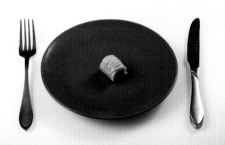

	CARBS	CALS	PROT	FAT
2x	18g	158	2g	8g
3x	27g	237	3g	12g
4x	36g	316	4g	16g
Weight: 20g				

| 13g CARBS | 110 CALS | 1g PROTEIN | 6g FAT |

	CARBS	CALS	PROT	FAT
2x	26g	220	2g	12g
3x	39g	330	3g	18g
4x	52g	440	4g	24g
Weight: 28g				

| 6g CARBS | 55 CALS | 1g PROTEIN | 3g FAT |

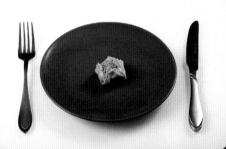

	CARBS	CALS	PROT	FAT
2x	12g	110	2g	6g
3x	18g	165	3g	9g
4x	24g	220	4g	12g
Weight: 14g				

| 12g CARBS | 102 CALS | 1g PROTEIN | 5g FAT |

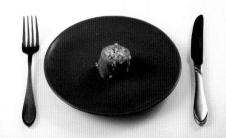

	CARBS	CALS	PROT	FAT
2x	24g	204	2g	10g
3x	36g	306	3g	15g
4x	48g	408	4g	20g
Weight: 26g				

Bakewell Tart

15g CARBS	155 CALS	2g PROTEIN	10g FAT

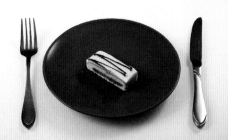

Weight: 34g

20g CARBS	205 CALS	3g PROTEIN	13g FAT

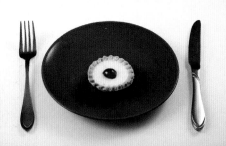

Weight: 45g

40g CARBS	424 CALS	6g PROTEIN	28g FAT

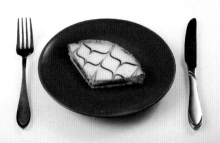

Weight: 93g

Carrot Cake

20g CARBS	190 CALS	2g PROTEIN	12g FAT

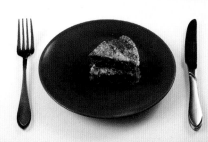

Weight: 53g

40g CARBS	384 CALS	5g PROTEIN	24g FAT

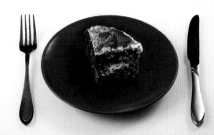

Weight: 107g

60g CARBS	578 CALS	7g PROTEIN	37g FAT

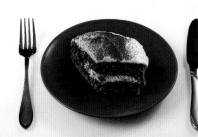

Weight: 161g

Chocolate Cake

20g CARBS	186 CALS	3g PROTEIN	11g FAT

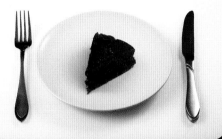

Weight: 40g

35g CARBS	325 CALS	5g PROTEIN	19g FAT

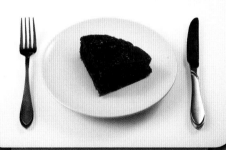

Weight: 70g

70g CARBS	640 CALS	10g PROTEIN	38g FAT

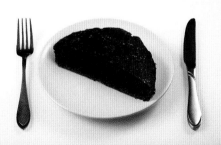

Weight: 138g

Fruit Cake

16g CARBS	89 CALS	1g PROTEIN	3g FAT

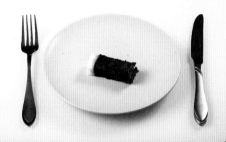

Weight: 26g

36g CARBS	206 CALS	2g PROTEIN	7g FAT

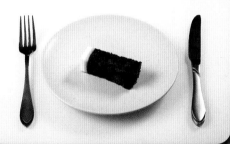

Weight: 60g

72g CARBS	415 CALS	5g PROTEIN	14g FAT

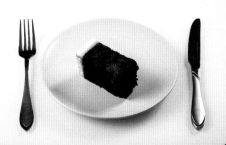

Weight: 121g

Ginger Cake

| 15g CARBS | 86 CALS | 1g PROTEIN | 3g FAT |

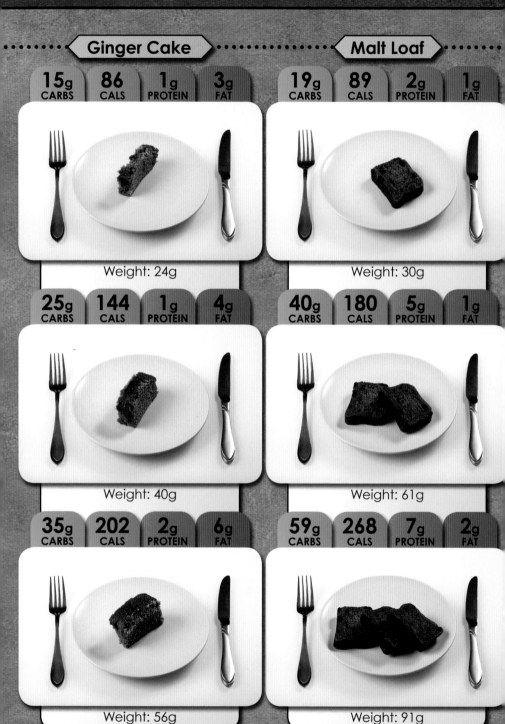

Weight: 24g

| 25g CARBS | 144 CALS | 1g PROTEIN | 4g FAT |

Weight: 40g

| 35g CARBS | 202 CALS | 2g PROTEIN | 6g FAT |

Weight: 56g

Malt Loaf

| 19g CARBS | 89 CALS | 2g PROTEIN | 1g FAT |

Weight: 30g

| 40g CARBS | 180 CALS | 5g PROTEIN | 1g FAT |

Weight: 61g

| 59g CARBS | 268 CALS | 7g PROTEIN | 2g FAT |

Weight: 91g

Swiss Roll

17g CARBS	134 CALS	2g PROTEIN	7g FAT

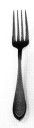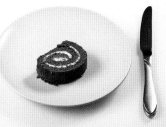

Weight: 35g

33g CARBS	264 CALS	3g PROTEIN	14g FAT

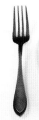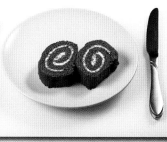

Weight: 69g

49g CARBS	394 CALS	5g PROTEIN	20g FAT

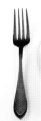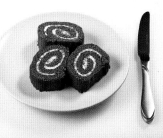

Weight: 103g

Victoria Sponge

19g CARBS	123 CALS	2g PROTEIN	5g FAT

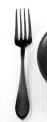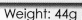

Weight: 44g

34g CARBS	216 CALS	3g PROTEIN	8g FAT

Weight: 77g

68g CARBS	434 CALS	7g PROTEIN	17g FAT

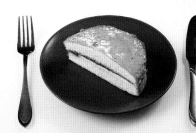

Weight: 155g

Apple Danish

| 45g CARBS | 298 CALS | 5g PROTEIN | 12g FAT |

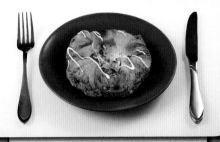

Weight: 87g

Choc Chip Twist

| 32g CARBS | 340 CALS | 4g PROTEIN | 22g FAT |

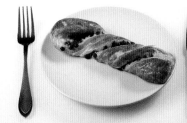

Weight: 85g

Cinnamon Swirl

| 41g CARBS | 270 CALS | 5g PROTEIN | 11g FAT |

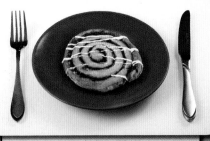

Weight: 79g

Fruit Trellis

| 28g CARBS | 206 CALS | 3g PROTEIN | 10g FAT |

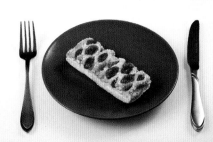

Weight: 58g

Pain au Raisin

| 44g CARBS | 364 CALS | 7g PROTEIN | 18g FAT |

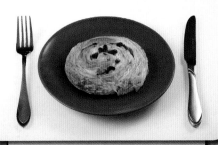

Weight: 95g

Pecan Plait

| 36g CARBS | 347 CALS | 5g PROTEIN | 21g FAT |

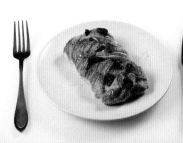

Weight: 81g

Chocolate Éclair

| 21g CARBS | 217 CALS | 2g PROTEIN | 14g FAT |

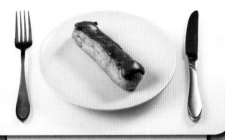

Weight: 56g

Corn Flake Cake

| 35g CARBS | 248 CALS | 4g PROTEIN | 10g FAT |

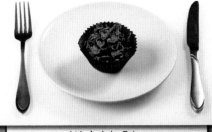

Weight: 54g

Cup Cake

| 34g CARBS | 272 CALS | 2g PROTEIN | 14g FAT |

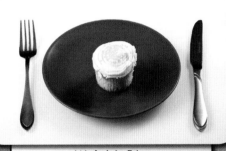

Weight: 56g

Custard Slice

| 40g CARBS | 286 CALS | 2g PROTEIN | 13g FAT |

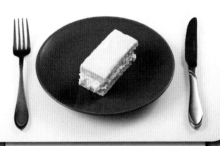

Weight: 106g

Custard Tart

| 26g CARBS | 263 CALS | 5g PROTEIN | 16g FAT |

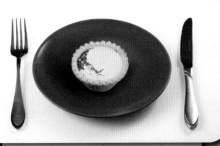

Weight: 92g

Mini Battenburg

| 16g CARBS | 112 CALS | 2g PROTEIN | 5g FAT |

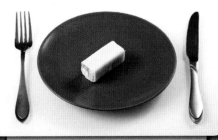

Weight: 30g

Choc Ring Doughnut

25g CARBS	201 CALS	2g PROTEIN	10g FAT

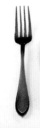
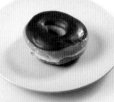
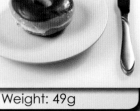

Weight: 49g

Glazed Ring Doughnut

25g CARBS	176 CALS	2g PROTEIN	8g FAT

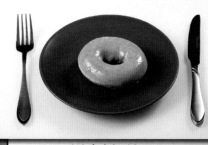

Weight: 46g

Jam Doughnut

35g CARBS	239 CALS	4g PROTEIN	10g FAT

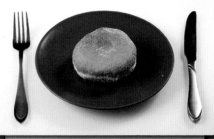
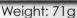

Weight: 71g

Mini Doughnut

6g CARBS	45 CALS	1g PROTEIN	2g FAT

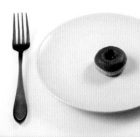

Weight: 11g

Sprinkle Ring Doughnut

32g CARBS	240 CALS	3g PROTEIN	11g FAT

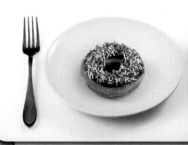
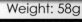

Weight: 58g

Sugar Ring Doughnut

31g CARBS	266 CALS	4g PROTEIN	15g FAT

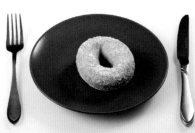

Weight: 66g

Fresh Cream Doughnut

25g CARBS	221 CALS	4g PROTEIN	12g FAT

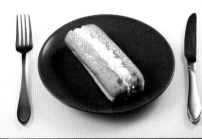

Weight: 69g

Yum Yum

32g CARBS	276 CALS	4g PROTEIN	15g FAT

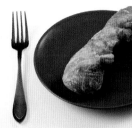

Weight: 70g

Blueberry Muffin

12g CARBS	86 CALS	1g PROTEIN	4g FAT

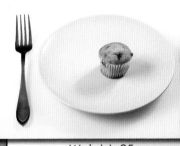
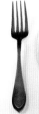

Weight: 25g

48g CARBS	353 CALS	6g PROTEIN	16g FAT

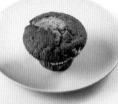

Weight: 102g

Chocolate Muffin

15g CARBS	108 CALS	2g PROTEIN	5g FAT

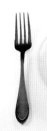
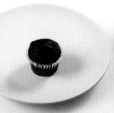
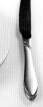

Weight: 28g

55g CARBS	404 CALS	7g PROTEIN	19g FAT

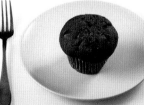
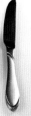

Weight: 105g

Flapjack

31g CARBS	**247** CALS	**2**g PROTEIN	**14**g FAT

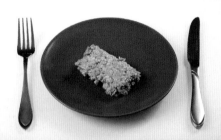

Weight: 50g

51g CARBS	**404** CALS	**4**g PROTEIN	**22**g FAT

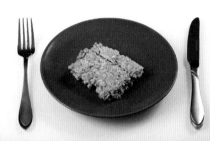

Weight: 82g

Meringue Nest

5g CARBS	**19** CALS	**0**g PROTEIN	**0**g FAT

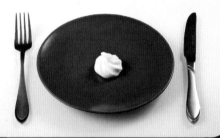

Weight: 5g

15g CARBS	**61** CALS	**1**g PROTEIN	**0**g FAT

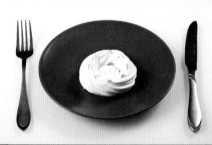

Weight: 16g

Mince Pie

25g CARBS	**183** CALS	**2**g PROTEIN	**9**g FAT

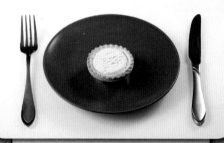

Weight: 42g

36g CARBS	**261** CALS	**3**g PROTEIN	**13**g FAT

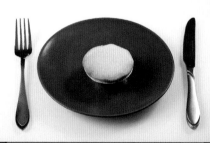

Weight: 60g

Belgian Bun

69g CARBS	411 CALS	6g PROTEIN	12g FAT

Weight: 116g

Cheese Scone

30g CARBS	251 CALS	7g PROTEIN	12g FAT

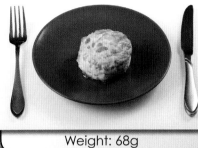

Weight: 68g

Fruit Scone

21g CARBS	120 CALS	2g PROTEIN	3g FAT

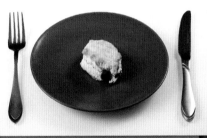

Weight: 38g

37g CARBS	208 CALS	4g PROTEIN	6g FAT

Weight: 66g

Hot Cross Bun

30g CARBS	159 CALS	4g PROTEIN	4g FAT

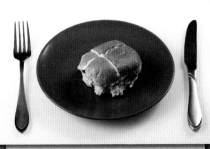

Weight: 51g

Iced Bun

20g CARBS	113 CALS	2g PROTEIN	3g FAT

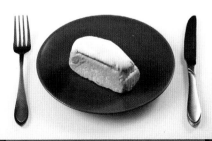

Weight: 37g

Apple Pie

18g CARBS	134 CALS	1g PROTEIN	7g FAT

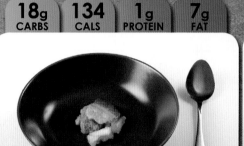

Weight: 50g

36g CARBS	267 CALS	3g PROTEIN	14g FAT

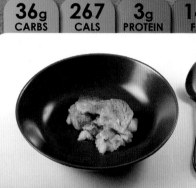

Weight: 100g

54g CARBS	403 CALS	4g PROTEIN	20g FAT

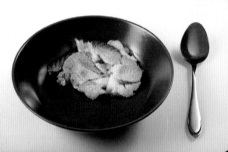

Weight: 151g

72g CARBS	537 CALS	6g PROTEIN	27g FAT

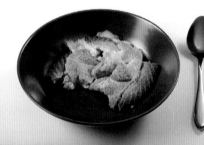

Weight: 201g

90g CARBS	673 CALS	7g PROTEIN	34g FAT

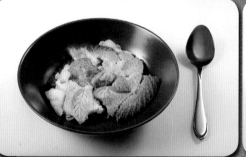

Weight: 252g

108g CARBS	806 CALS	9g PROTEIN	41g FAT

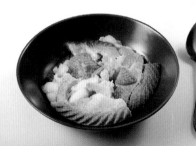

Weight: 302g

Apple & Rhubarb Crumble

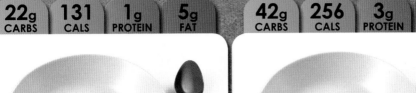

22g CARBS	131 CALS	1g PROTEIN	5g FAT

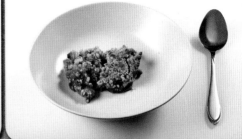

Weight: 60g

42g CARBS	256 CALS	3g PROTEIN	10g FAT

Weight: 117g

63g CARBS	383 CALS	4g PROTEIN	15g FAT

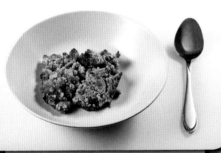

Weight: 175g

85g CARBS	515 CALS	6g PROTEIN	20g FAT

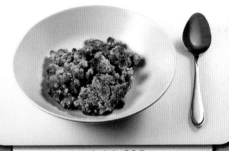

Weight: 235g

106g CARBS	646 CALS	7g PROTEIN	24g FAT

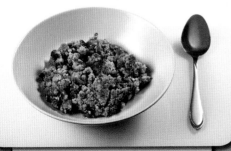

Weight: 295g

127g CARBS	771 CALS	8g PROTEIN	29g FAT

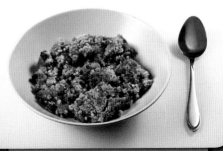

Weight: 352g

Apple Strudel

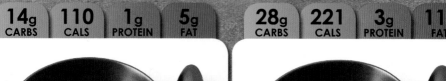

| 14g CARBS | 110 CALS | 1g PROTEIN | 5g FAT |

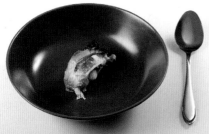

Weight: 45g

| 28g CARBS | 221 CALS | 3g PROTEIN | 11g FAT |

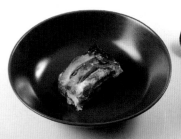

Weight: 90g

| 42g CARBS | 331 CALS | 4g PROTEIN | 16g FAT |

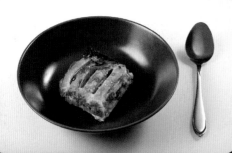

Weight: 135g

| 56g CARBS | 446 CALS | 5g PROTEIN | 22g FAT |

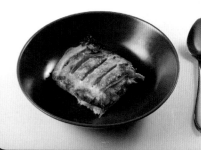

Weight: 182g

| 70g CARBS | 559 CALS | 7g PROTEIN | 27g FAT |

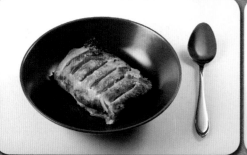

Weight: 228g

| 84g CARBS | 666 CALS | 8g PROTEIN | 33g FAT |

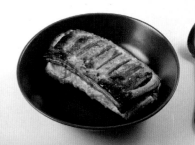

Weight: 272g

Banoffee Pie

14g CARBS	137 CALS	2g PROTEIN	9g FAT

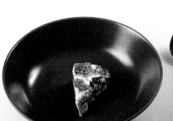

Weight: 43g

29g CARBS	284 CALS	3g PROTEIN	18g FAT

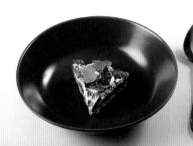

Weight: 89g

44g CARBS	424 CALS	5g PROTEIN	27g FAT

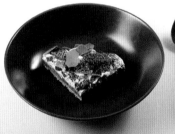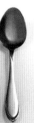

Weight: 133g

58g CARBS	561 CALS	7g PROTEIN	35g FAT

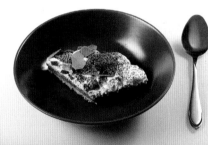

Weight: 176g

72g CARBS	702 CALS	8g PROTEIN	44g FAT

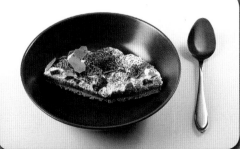

Weight: 220g

87g CARBS	845 CALS	10g PROTEIN	53g FAT

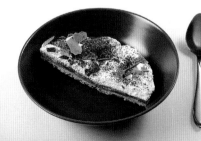

Weight: 265g

Black Forest Gateau

13g CARBS	103 CALS	1g PROTEIN	5g FAT

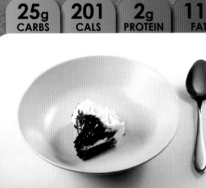

Weight: 35g

25g CARBS	201 CALS	2g PROTEIN	11g FAT

Weight: 68g

37g CARBS	295 CALS	4g PROTEIN	16g FAT

Weight: 100g

50g CARBS	398 CALS	5g PROTEIN	21g FAT

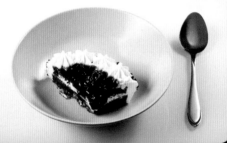

Weight: 135g

62g CARBS	496 CALS	6g PROTEIN	26g FAT

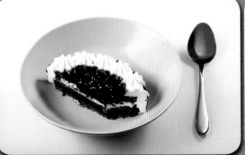

Weight: 168g

74g CARBS	590 CALS	7g PROTEIN	31g FAT

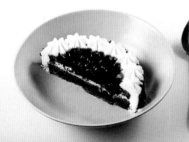

Weight: 200g

Bread & Butter Pudding

10g CARBS	**98** CALS	**2g** PROTEIN	**5g** FAT

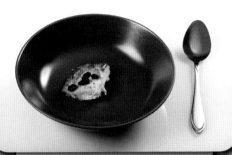

Weight: 40g

19g CARBS	**199** CALS	**5g** PROTEIN	**11g** FAT

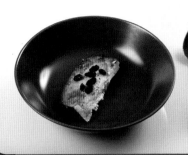

Weight: 81g

29g CARBS	**300** CALS	**7g** PROTEIN	**16g** FAT

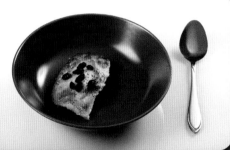

Weight: 122g

39g CARBS	**403** CALS	**9g** PROTEIN	**22g** FAT

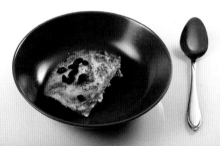

Weight: 164g

49g CARBS	**504** CALS	**11g** PROTEIN	**28g** FAT

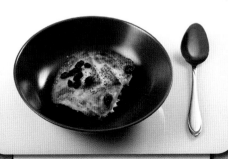

Weight: 205g

59g CARBS	**605** CALS	**14g** PROTEIN	**33g** FAT

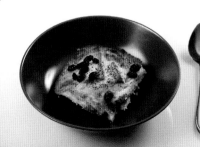

Weight: 246g

Brownie

24g CARBS	199 CALS	2g PROTEIN	11g FAT

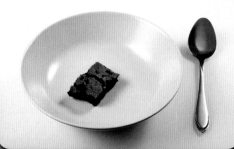

Weight: 45g

43g CARBS	362 CALS	4g PROTEIN	20g FAT

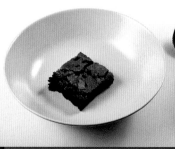

Weight: 82g

67g CARBS	561 CALS	6g PROTEIN	31g FAT

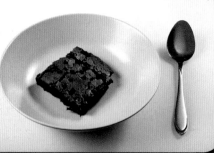

Weight: 127g

87g CARBS	725 CALS	8g PROTEIN	40g FAT

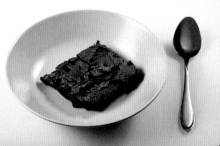

Weight: 164g

111g CARBS	924 CALS	10g PROTEIN	51g FAT

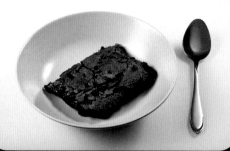

Weight: 209g

130g CARBS	1087 CALS	12g PROTEIN	60g FAT

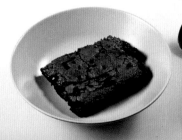

Weight: 246g

Cheesecake

18g CARBS	147 CALS	2g PROTEIN	8g FAT

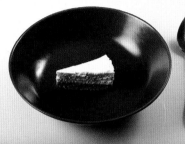

Weight: 50g

35g CARBS	294 CALS	4g PROTEIN	16g FAT

Weight: 100g

53g CARBS	441 CALS	6g PROTEIN	24g FAT

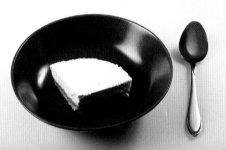

Weight: 150g

70g CARBS	588 CALS	8g PROTEIN	32g FAT

Weight: 200g

88g CARBS	735 CALS	10g PROTEIN	41g FAT

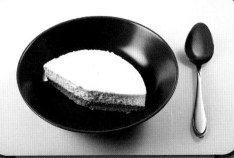

Weight: 250g

106g CARBS	882 CALS	12g PROTEIN	49g FAT

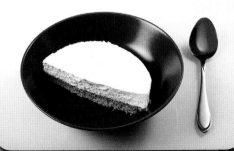

Weight: 300g

Chocolate Torte

11g CARBS	140 CALS	2g PROTEIN	10g FAT

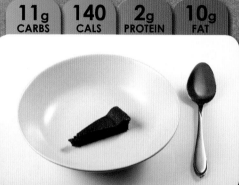

Weight: 33g

21g CARBS	279 CALS	4g PROTEIN	20g FAT

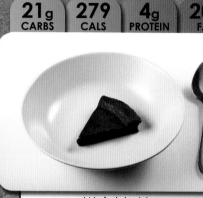

Weight: 66g

32g CARBS	423 CALS	6g PROTEIN	30g FAT

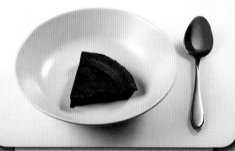

Weight: 100g

43g CARBS	563 CALS	8g PROTEIN	40g FAT

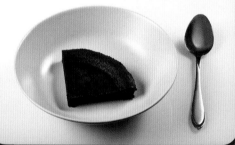

Weight: 133g

53g CARBS	702 CALS	9g PROTEIN	50g FAT

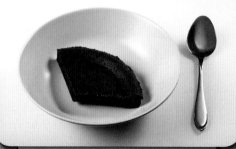

Weight: 166g

64g CARBS	846 CALS	11g PROTEIN	60g FAT

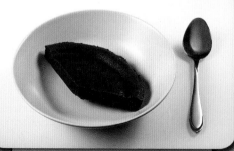

Weight: 200g

Christmas Pudding

| 20g CARBS | 115 CALS | 1g PROTEIN | 4g FAT |

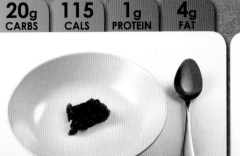

Weight: 35g

| 40g CARBS | 234 CALS | 2g PROTEIN | 8g FAT |

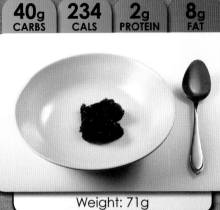

Weight: 71g

| 60g CARBS | 349 CALS | 3g PROTEIN | 13g FAT |

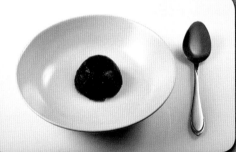

Weight: 106g (individual)

| 80g CARBS | 467 CALS | 4g PROTEIN | 17g FAT |

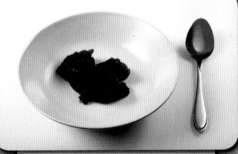

Weight: 142g

| 100g CARBS | 582 CALS | 5g PROTEIN | 21g FAT |

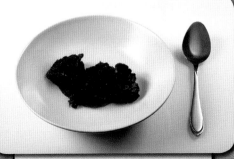

Weight: 177g

| 120g CARBS | 704 CALS | 6g PROTEIN | 25g FAT |

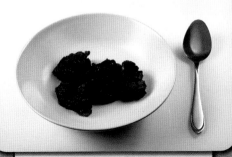

Weight: 214g

Custard (made with whole milk)

10g CARBS	71 CALS	2g PROTEIN	3g FAT

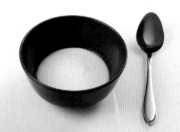

Weight: 60g

19g CARBS	142 CALS	5g PROTEIN	5g FAT

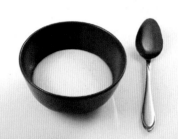

Weight: 120g

29g CARBS	212 CALS	7g PROTEIN	8g FAT

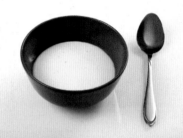

Weight: 180g

39g CARBS	283 CALS	9g PROTEIN	11g FAT

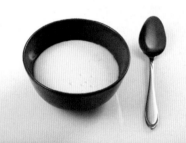

Weight: 240g

49g CARBS	354 CALS	12g PROTEIN	14g FAT

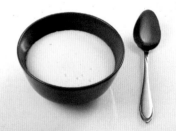

Weight: 300g

58g CARBS	425 CALS	14g PROTEIN	16g FAT

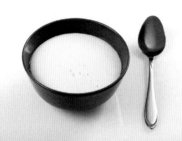

Weight: 360g

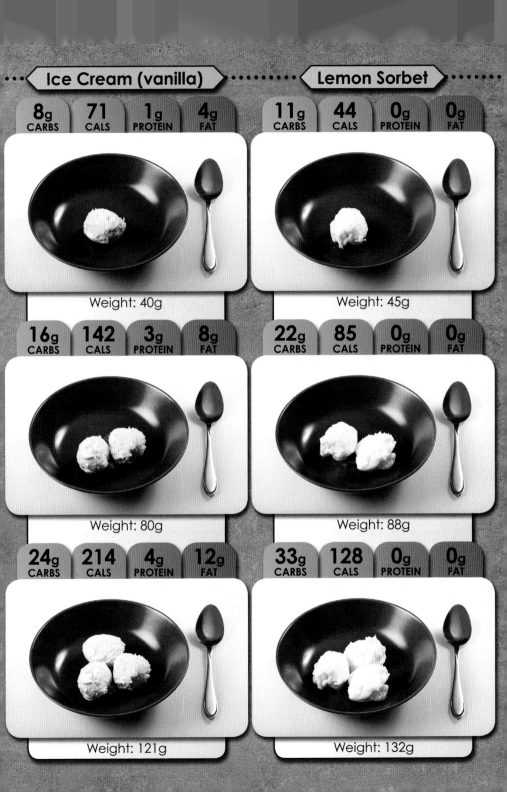

Ice Cream (vanilla)

| 8g CARBS | 71 CALS | 1g PROTEIN | 4g FAT |

Weight: 40g

| 16g CARBS | 142 CALS | 3g PROTEIN | 8g FAT |

Weight: 80g

| 24g CARBS | 214 CALS | 4g PROTEIN | 12g FAT |

Weight: 121g

Lemon Sorbet

| 11g CARBS | 44 CALS | 0g PROTEIN | 0g FAT |

Weight: 45g

| 22g CARBS | 85 CALS | 0g PROTEIN | 0g FAT |

Weight: 88g

| 33g CARBS | 128 CALS | 0g PROTEIN | 0g FAT |

Weight: 132g

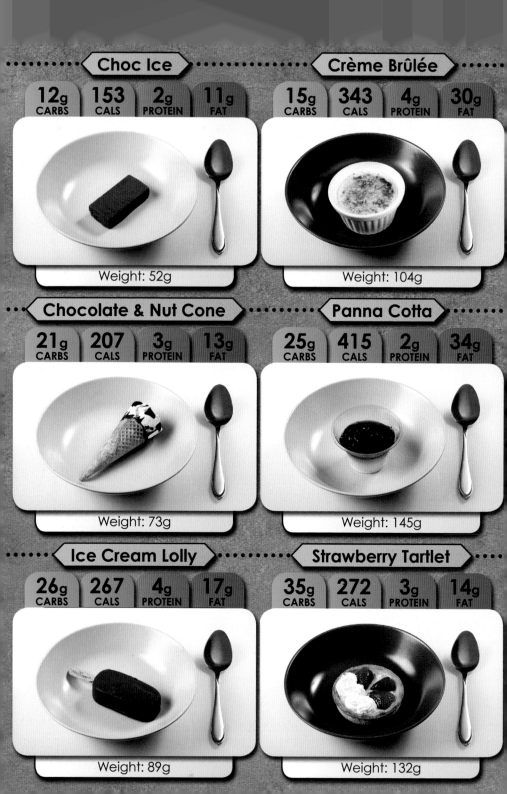

Choc Ice

| 12g CARBS | 153 CALS | 2g PROTEIN | 11g FAT |

Weight: 52g

Crème Brûlée

| 15g CARBS | 343 CALS | 4g PROTEIN | 30g FAT |

Weight: 104g

Chocolate & Nut Cone

| 21g CARBS | 207 CALS | 3g PROTEIN | 13g FAT |

Weight: 73g

Panna Cotta

| 25g CARBS | 415 CALS | 2g PROTEIN | 34g FAT |

Weight: 145g

Ice Cream Lolly

| 26g CARBS | 267 CALS | 4g PROTEIN | 17g FAT |

Weight: 89g

Strawberry Tartlet

| 35g CARBS | 272 CALS | 3g PROTEIN | 14g FAT |

Weight: 132g

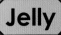

Jelly

10g CARBS	40 CALS	1g PROTEIN	0g FAT

Weight: 65g

20g CARBS	79 CALS	2g PROTEIN	0g FAT

Weight: 130g

30g CARBS	122 CALS	2g PROTEIN	0g FAT

Weight: 200g

40g CARBS	162 CALS	3g PROTEIN	0g FAT

Weight: 265g

50g CARBS	201 CALS	4g PROTEIN	0g FAT

Weight: 330g

60g CARBS	244 CALS	5g PROTEIN	0g FAT

Weight: 400g

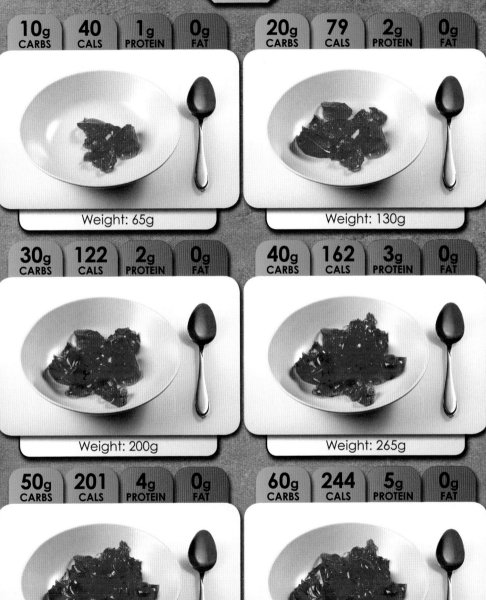

Lemon Meringue Pie

| 19g CARBS | 110 CALS | 1g PROTEIN | 4g FAT |

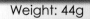

Weight: 44g

| 38g CARBS | 221 CALS | 3g PROTEIN | 7g FAT |

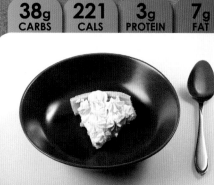

Weight: 88g

| 57g CARBS | 326 CALS | 4g PROTEIN | 11g FAT |

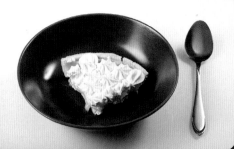

Weight: 130g

| 76g CARBS | 439 CALS | 5g PROTEIN | 15g FAT |

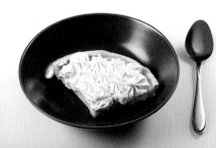

Weight: 175g

| 95g CARBS | 547 CALS | 6g PROTEIN | 19g FAT |

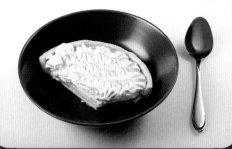

Weight: 218g

| 114g CARBS | 658 CALS | 8g PROTEIN | 22g FAT |

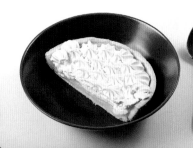

Weight: 262g

Mousse (chocolate)

10g CARBS	75 CALS	2g PROTEIN	3g FAT

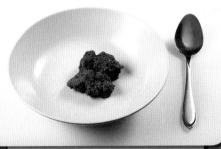

Weight: 50g

20g CARBS	149 CALS	4g PROTEIN	7g FAT

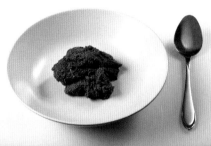

Weight: 100g

30g CARBS	224 CALS	6g PROTEIN	10g FAT

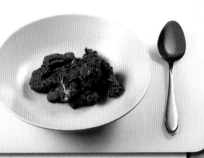

Weight: 150g

40g CARBS	298 CALS	8g PROTEIN	13g FAT

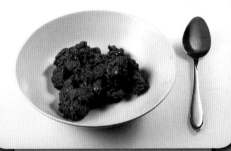

Weight: 200g

50g CARBS	373 CALS	10g PROTEIN	16g FAT

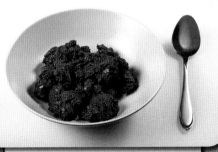

Weight: 250g

60g CARBS	447 CALS	12g PROTEIN	20g FAT

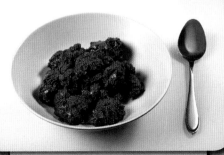

Weight: 300g

Profiteroles

10g CARBS	138 CALS	2g PROTEIN	10g FAT

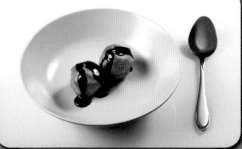

Weight: 40g

20g CARBS	277 CALS	4g PROTEIN	21g FAT

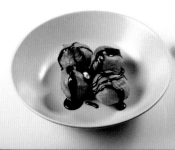

Weight: 80g

30g CARBS	415 CALS	7g PROTEIN	31g FAT

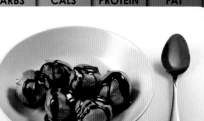

Weight: 120g

40g CARBS	557 CALS	9g PROTEIN	41g FAT

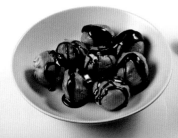

Weight: 161g

50g CARBS	709 CALS	11g PROTEIN	53g FAT

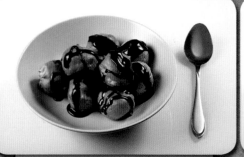

Weight: 205g

60g CARBS	848 CALS	13g PROTEIN	63g FAT

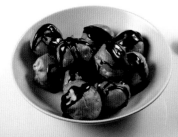

Weight: 245g

Rice Pudding

11g CARBS	60 CALS	2g PROTEIN	1g FAT

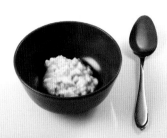

Weight: 70g

23g CARBS	119 CALS	5g PROTEIN	2g FAT

Weight: 140g

35g CARBS	183 CALS	7g PROTEIN	3g FAT

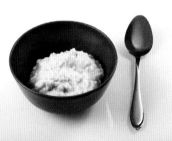

Weight: 215g

46g CARBS	242 CALS	9g PROTEIN	4g FAT

Weight: 285g

57g CARBS	302 CALS	12g PROTEIN	5g FAT

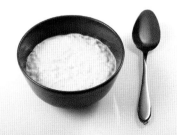

Weight: 355g

68g CARBS	361 CALS	14g PROTEIN	6g FAT

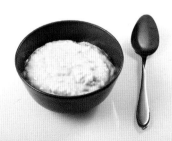

Weight: 425g

Roulade

| 18g CARBS | 154 CALS | 1g PROTEIN | 9g FAT |

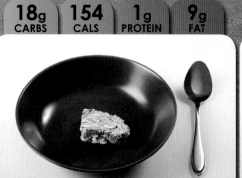

Weight: 38g

| 36g CARBS | 308 CALS | 3g PROTEIN | 17g FAT |

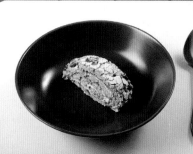

Weight: 76g

| 54g CARBS | 462 CALS | 4g PROTEIN | 26g FAT |

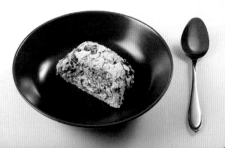

Weight: 114g

| 72g CARBS | 624 CALS | 6g PROTEIN | 34g FAT |

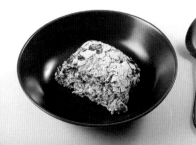

Weight: 154g

| 90g CARBS | 778 CALS | 7g PROTEIN | 43g FAT |

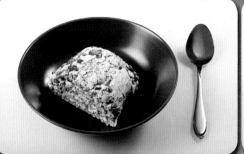

Weight: 192g

| 108g CARBS | 932 CALS | 9g PROTEIN | 52g FAT |

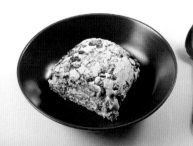

Weight: 230g

Spotted Dick

25g CARBS	180 CALS	2g PROTEIN	9g FAT

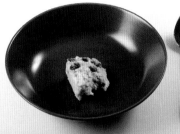

Weight: 52g

50g CARBS	363 CALS	5g PROTEIN	17g FAT

Weight: 105g (individual)

75g CARBS	547 CALS	8g PROTEIN	26g FAT

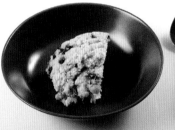

Weight: 158g

100g CARBS	730 CALS	10g PROTEIN	35g FAT

Weight: 211g

125g CARBS	913 CALS	13g PROTEIN	44g FAT

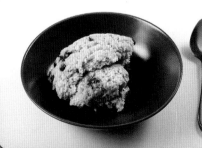

Weight: 264g

150g CARBS	1097 CALS	15g PROTEIN	53g FAT

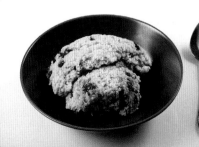

Weight: 317g

Sticky Toffee Pudding

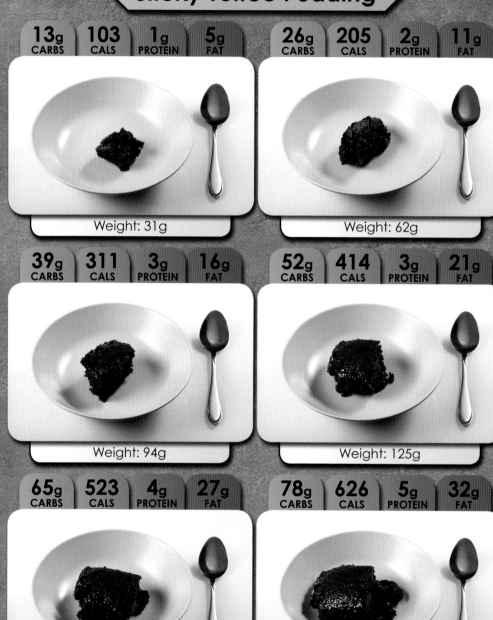

| 13g CARBS | 103 CALS | 1g PROTEIN | 5g FAT |
Weight: 31g

| 26g CARBS | 205 CALS | 2g PROTEIN | 11g FAT |
Weight: 62g

| 39g CARBS | 311 CALS | 3g PROTEIN | 16g FAT |
Weight: 94g

| 52g CARBS | 414 CALS | 3g PROTEIN | 21g FAT |
Weight: 125g

| 65g CARBS | 523 CALS | 4g PROTEIN | 27g FAT |
Weight: 158g

| 78g CARBS | 626 CALS | 5g PROTEIN | 32g FAT |
Weight: 189g

Strawberry Delight

5g CARBS	38 CALS	1g PROTEIN	2g FAT

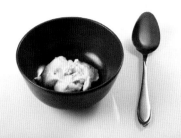

Weight: 33g

15g CARBS	116 CALS	3g PROTEIN	5g FAT

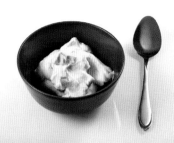

Weight: 100g

25g CARBS	193 CALS	5g PROTEIN	8g FAT

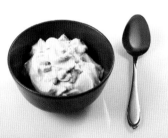

Weight: 166g

35g CARBS	270 CALS	8g PROTEIN	11g FAT

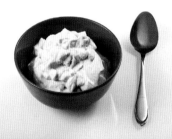

Weight: 233g

45g CARBS	348 CALS	10g PROTEIN	14g FAT

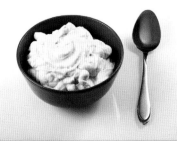

Weight: 300g

56g CARBS	427 CALS	12g PROTEIN	18g FAT

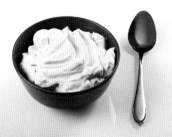

Weight: 368g

Summer Pudding

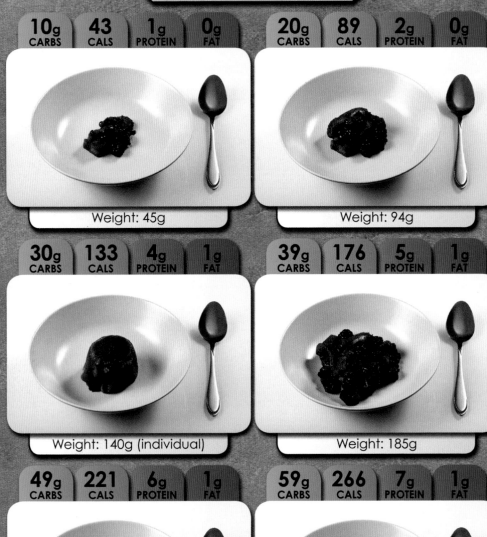

10g CARBS	43 CALS	1g PROTEIN	0g FAT

Weight: 45g

20g CARBS	89 CALS	2g PROTEIN	0g FAT

Weight: 94g

30g CARBS	133 CALS	4g PROTEIN	1g FAT

Weight: 140g (individual)

39g CARBS	176 CALS	5g PROTEIN	1g FAT

Weight: 185g

49g CARBS	221 CALS	6g PROTEIN	1g FAT

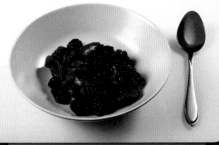

Weight: 233g

59g CARBS	266 CALS	7g PROTEIN	1g FAT

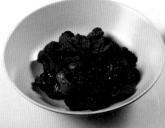

Weight: 280g

Tiramisu

15g CARBS	119 CALS	2g PROTEIN	5g FAT

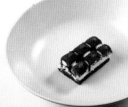

Weight: 45g

30g CARBS	239 CALS	4g PROTEIN	11g FAT

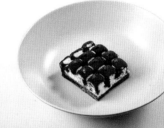

Weight: 90g

45g CARBS	355 CALS	6g PROTEIN	16g FAT

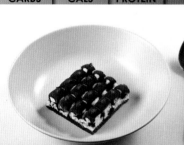

Weight: 134g

59g CARBS	472 CALS	9g PROTEIN	22g FAT

Weight: 178g

74g CARBS	588 CALS	11g PROTEIN	27g FAT

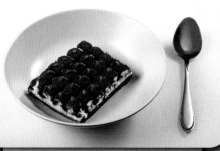

Weight: 222g

89g CARBS	702 CALS	13g PROTEIN	32g FAT

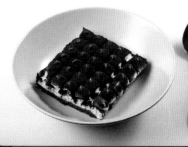

Weight: 265g

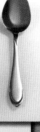
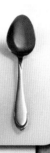

| 12g CARBS | 91 CALS | 1g PROTEIN | 4g FAT |

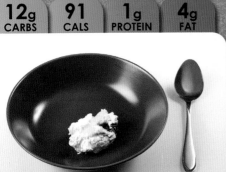
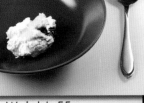

Weight: 55g

| 23g CARBS | 178 CALS | 3g PROTEIN | 9g FAT |

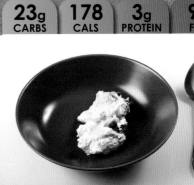

Weight: 108g

| 34g CARBS | 267 CALS | 4g PROTEIN | 13g FAT |

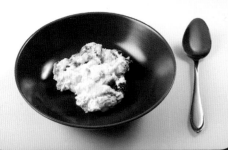

Weight: 162g

| 45g CARBS | 355 CALS | 6g PROTEIN | 17g FAT |

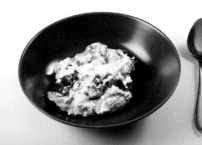

Weight: 215g

| 57g CARBS | 446 CALS | 7g PROTEIN | 22g FAT |

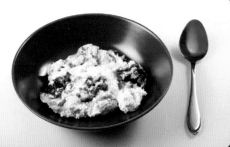

Weight: 270g

| 68g CARBS | 536 CALS | 8g PROTEIN | 26g FAT |

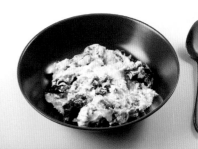

Weight: 325g

Apple Juice

| 16g CARBS | 61 CALS | 0g PROTEIN | 0g FAT |

160ml

| 28g CARBS | 109 CALS | 0g PROTEIN | 0g FAT |

284ml (half pint)

| 57g CARBS | 218 CALS | 1g PROTEIN | 1g FAT |

568ml (pint)

Cranberry Juice

| 23g CARBS | 98 CALS | 0g PROTEIN | 0g FAT |

160ml

| 41g CARBS | 175 CALS | 0g PROTEIN | 0g FAT |

284ml (half pint)

| 83g CARBS | 350 CALS | 0g PROTEIN | 0g FAT |

568ml (pint)

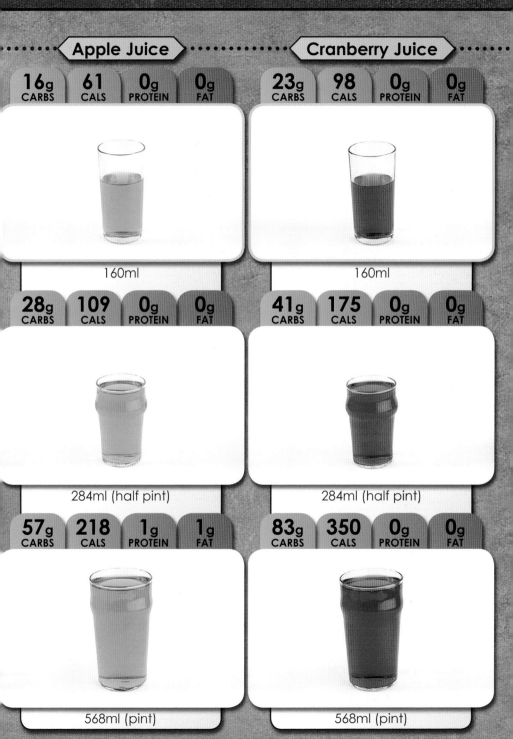

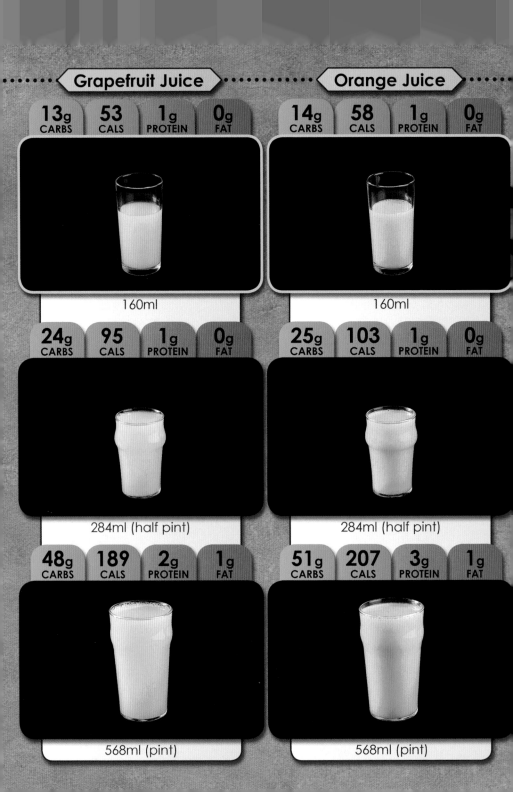

Grapefruit Juice

| 13g CARBS | 53 CALS | 1g PROTEIN | 0g FAT |

160ml

| 24g CARBS | 95 CALS | 1g PROTEIN | 0g FAT |

284ml (half pint)

| 48g CARBS | 189 CALS | 2g PROTEIN | 1g FAT |

568ml (pint)

Orange Juice

| 14g CARBS | 58 CALS | 1g PROTEIN | 0g FAT |

160ml

| 25g CARBS | 103 CALS | 1g PROTEIN | 0g FAT |

284ml (half pint)

| 51g CARBS | 207 CALS | 3g PROTEIN | 1g FAT |

568ml (pint)

Pineapple Juice

| 17g CARBS | 66 CALS | 0g PROTEIN | 0g FAT |

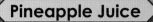

160ml

| 30g CARBS | 118 CALS | 1g PROTEIN | 0g FAT |

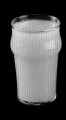

284ml (half pint)

| 60g CARBS | 235 CALS | 2g PROTEIN | 1g FAT |

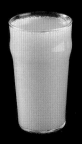

568ml (pint)

Tomato Juice

| 5g CARBS | 22 CALS | 1g PROTEIN | 0g FAT |

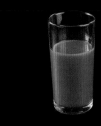

160ml

| 9g CARBS | 40 CALS | 2g PROTEIN | 0g FAT |

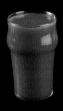

284ml (half pint)

| 17g CARBS | 80 CALS | 5g PROTEIN | 0g FAT |

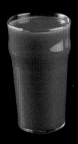

568ml (pint)

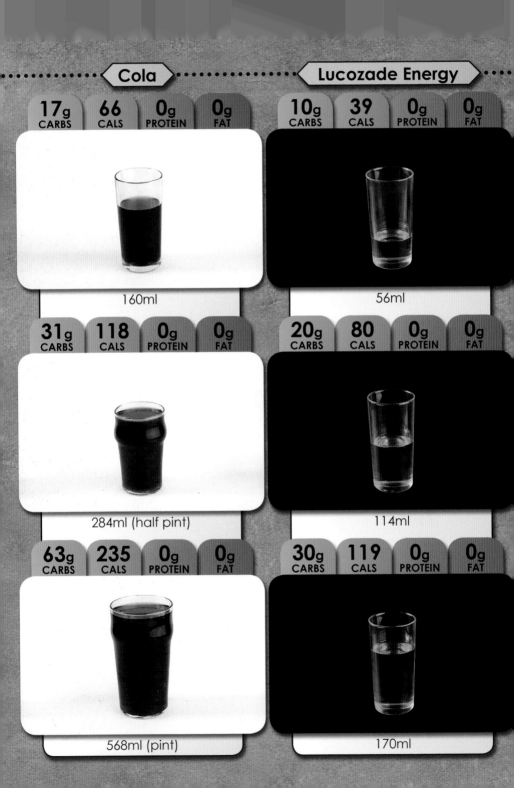

Cola

| 17g CARBS | 66 CALS | 0g PROTEIN | 0g FAT |

160ml

| 31g CARBS | 118 CALS | 0g PROTEIN | 0g FAT |

284ml (half pint)

| 63g CARBS | 235 CALS | 0g PROTEIN | 0g FAT |

568ml (pint)

Lucozade Energy

| 10g CARBS | 39 CALS | 0g PROTEIN | 0g FAT |

56ml

| 20g CARBS | 80 CALS | 0g PROTEIN | 0g FAT |

114ml

| 30g CARBS | 119 CALS | 0g PROTEIN | 0g FAT |

170ml

Milk (skimmed)

7g CARBS	51 CALS	5g PROTEIN	0g FAT

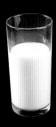

160ml

13g CARBS	92 CALS	10g PROTEIN	1g FAT

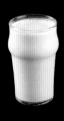

284ml (half pint)

25g CARBS	184 CALS	20g PROTEIN	1g FAT

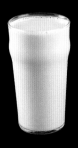

568ml (pint)

Milk (semi-skimmed)

8g CARBS	74 CALS	5g PROTEIN	3g FAT

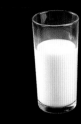

160ml

13g CARBS	132 CALS	10g PROTEIN	5g FAT

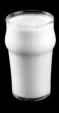

284ml (half pint)

27g CARBS	264 CALS	20g PROTEIN	10g FAT

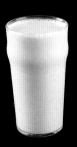

568ml (pint)

Milk (whole)

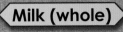

7g CARBS	106 CALS	5g PROTEIN	6g FAT

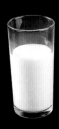

160ml

13g CARBS	189 CALS	9g PROTEIN	11g FAT

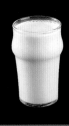

284ml (half pint)

26g CARBS	379 CALS	19g PROTEIN	22g FAT

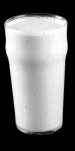

568ml (pint)

Soya Milk (sweetened)

4g CARBS	69 CALS	5g PROTEIN	4g FAT

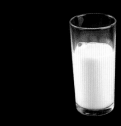

160ml

7g CARBS	123 CALS	9g PROTEIN	7g FAT

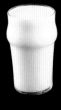

284ml (half pint)

14g CARBS	247 CALS	18g PROTEIN	14g FAT

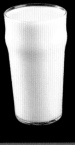

568ml (pint)

Fruit Smoothie (strawberry & banana)

| **20**g CARBS | **84** CALS | **1**g PROTEIN | **0**g FAT |

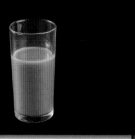

160ml

| **73**g CARBS | **302** CALS | **2**g PROTEIN | **1**g FAT |

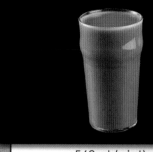

568ml (pint)

Milkshake (made with powder & semi-skimmed milk)

| **32**g CARBS | **198** CALS | **9**g PROTEIN | **5**g FAT |

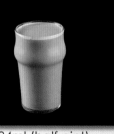

284ml (half pint)

| **65**g CARBS | **396** CALS | **18**g PROTEIN | **9**g FAT |

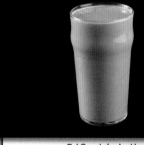

568ml (pint)

Hot Chocolate

| **28**g CARBS | **190** CALS | **9**g PROTEIN | **5**g FAT |

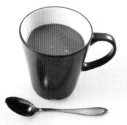

260ml

Hot Malt Drink

| **34**g CARBS | **221** CALS | **11**g PROTEIN | **5**g FAT |

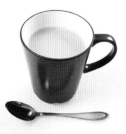

260ml

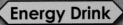

Energy Drink

13g CARBS	55 CALS	0g PROTEIN	0g FAT

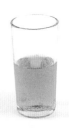

125ml (half can)

27g CARBS	111 CALS	0g PROTEIN	0g FAT

250ml (full can)

WKD

35g CARBS	207 CALS	0g PROTEIN	0g FAT

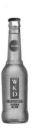

	CARBS	CALS	PROT	FAT
2x	70g	414	0g	0g
3x	105g	621	0g	0g
4x	140g	828	0g	0g

275ml bottle

WKD Core (cider)

47g CARBS	325 CALS	0g PROTEIN	0g FAT

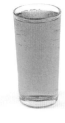

	CARBS	CALS	PROT	FAT
2x	94g	650	0g	0g
3x	141g	975	0g	0g
4x	188g	1300	0g	0g

500ml bottle

Lager (draught)

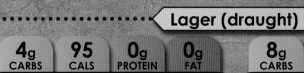

4g CARBS	**95** CALS	**0**g PROTEIN	**0**g FAT

284ml (half pint)

8g CARBS	**189** CALS	**0**g PROTEIN	**0**g FAT

568ml (pint)

Ale

9g CARBS	**86** CALS	**1**g PROTEIN	**0**g FAT

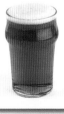

284ml (half pint)

17g CARBS	**172** CALS	**2**g PROTEIN	**0**g FAT

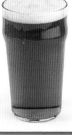

568ml (pint)

Stout

4g CARBS	**86** CALS	**1**g PROTEIN	**0**g FAT

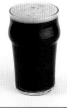

284ml (half pint)

9g CARBS	**172** CALS	**2**g PROTEIN	**0**g FAT

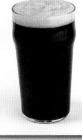

568ml (pint)

Cider (dry)

7g	103	0g	0g
CARBS	CALS	PROTEIN	FAT

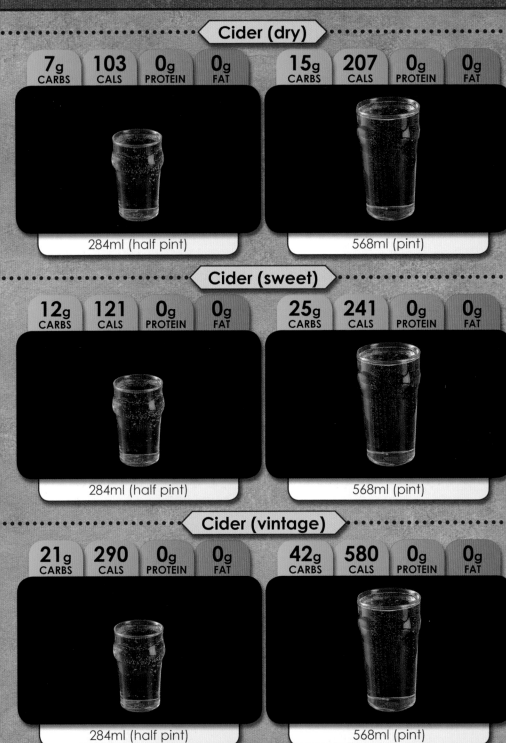

284ml (half pint)

15g	207	0g	0g
CARBS	CALS	PROTEIN	FAT

568ml (pint)

Cider (sweet)

12g	121	0g	0g
CARBS	CALS	PROTEIN	FAT

284ml (half pint)

25g	241	0g	0g
CARBS	CALS	PROTEIN	FAT

568ml (pint)

Cider (vintage)

21g	290	0g	0g
CARBS	CALS	PROTEIN	FAT

284ml (half pint)

42g	580	0g	0g
CARBS	CALS	PROTEIN	FAT

568ml (pint)

Red Wine

0g CARBS	85 CALS	0g PROTEIN	0g FAT

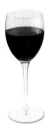

	CARBS	CALS	PROT	FAT
2x	0g	170	0g	0g
3x	0g	255	0g	0g
4x	0g	340	0g	0g
125ml (small glass)				

1g CARBS	170 CALS	0g PROTEIN	0g FAT

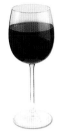

	CARBS	CALS	PROT	FAT
2x	2g	340	0g	0g
3x	3g	510	0g	0g
4x	4g	680	0g	0g
250ml (large glass)				

White Wine (dry)

1g CARBS	83 CALS	0g PROTEIN	0g FAT

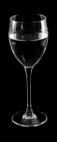

	CARBS	CALS	PROT	FAT
2x	2g	166	0g	0g
3x	3g	249	0g	0g
4x	4g	332	0g	0g
125ml (small glass)				

2g CARBS	165 CALS	0g PROTEIN	0g FAT

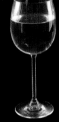

	CARBS	CALS	PROT	FAT
2x	4g	330	0g	0g
3x	6g	495	0g	0g
4x	8g	660	0g	0g
250ml (large glass)				

White Wine (sweet)

7g CARBS	**118** CALS	**0**g PROTEIN	**0**g FAT

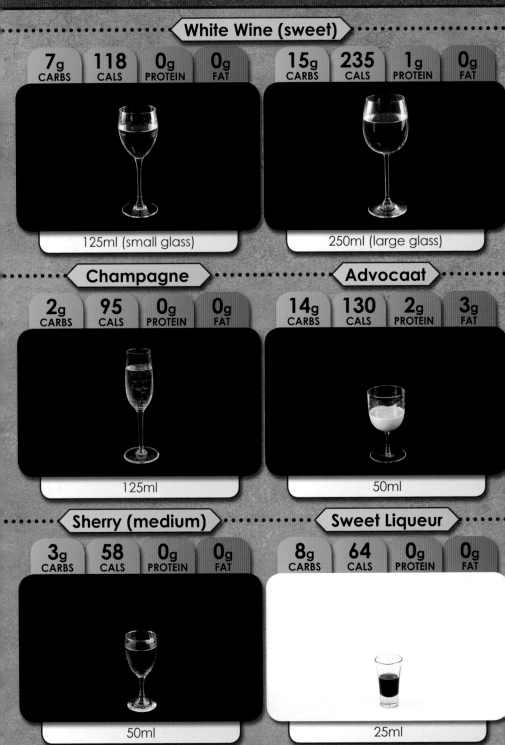

125ml (small glass)

15g CARBS	**235** CALS	**1**g PROTEIN	**0**g FAT

250ml (large glass)

Champagne

2g CARBS	**95** CALS	**0**g PROTEIN	**0**g FAT

125ml

Advocaat

14g CARBS	**130** CALS	**2**g PROTEIN	**3**g FAT

50ml

Sherry (medium)

3g CARBS	**58** CALS	**0**g PROTEIN	**0**g FAT

50ml

Sweet Liqueur

8g CARBS	**64** CALS	**0**g PROTEIN	**0**g FAT

25ml

Brandy

| 0g CARBS | 56 CALS | 0g PROTEIN | 0g FAT |

	CARBS	CALS	PROT	FAT
2x	0g	112	0g	0g
3x	0g	168	0g	0g
4x	0g	224	0g	0g
25ml

Irish Cream

| 12g CARBS | 163 CALS | 0g PROTEIN | 8g FAT |

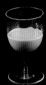

	CARBS	CALS	PROT	FAT
2x	24g	326	0g	16g
3x	36g	489	0g	24g
4x	48g	652	0g	32g
50ml

Port

| 6g CARBS | 79 CALS | 0g PROTEIN | 0g FAT |

	CARBS	CALS	PROT	FAT
2x	12g	158	0g	0g
3x	18g	237	0g	0g
4x	24g	316	0g	0g
50ml

Vermouth (sweet)

| 8g CARBS | 76 CALS | 0g PROTEIN | 0g FAT |

	CARBS	CALS	PROT	FAT
2x	16g	152	0g	0g
3x	24g	228	0g	0g
4x	32g	304	0g	0g
50ml

Gin

| 0g CARBS | 56 CALS | 0g PROTEIN | 0g FAT |

	CARBS	CALS	PROT	FAT
2x	0g	112	0g	0g
3x	0g	168	0g	0g
4x	0g	224	0g	0g
25ml				

Rum

| 0g CARBS | 56 CALS | 0g PROTEIN | 0g FAT |

	CARBS	CALS	PROT	FAT
2x	0g	112	0g	0g
3x	0g	168	0g	0g
4x	0g	224	0g	0g
25ml				

Vodka

| 0g CARBS | 56 CALS | 0g PROTEIN | 0g FAT |

	CARBS	CALS	PROT	FAT
2x	0g	112	0g	0g
3x	0g	168	0g	0g
4x	0g	224	0g	0g
25ml				

Whisky

| 0g CARBS | 56 CALS | 0g PROTEIN | 0g FAT |

	CARBS	CALS	PROT	FAT
2x	0g	112	0g	0g
3x	0g	168	0g	0g
4x	0g	224	0g	0g
25ml				

Boiled Egg

0g CARBS	88 CALS	8g PROTEIN	6g FAT

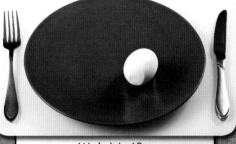

Weight: 60g

Scrambled Egg (with milk)

0g CARBS	154 CALS	7g PROTEIN	14g FAT

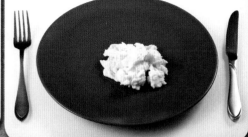

Weight: 60g (1 egg)

Fried Egg

0g CARBS	90 CALS	7g PROTEIN	7g FAT

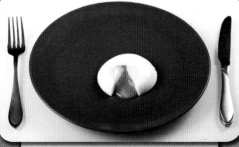

Weight: 50g

1g CARBS	308 CALS	13g PROTEIN	28g FAT

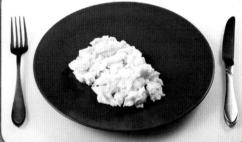

Weight: 120g (2 eggs)

Poached Egg

0g CARBS	74 CALS	6g PROTEIN	5g FAT

Weight: 50g

1g CARBS	463 CALS	20g PROTEIN	42g FAT

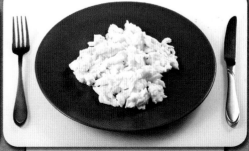

Weight: 180g (3 eggs)

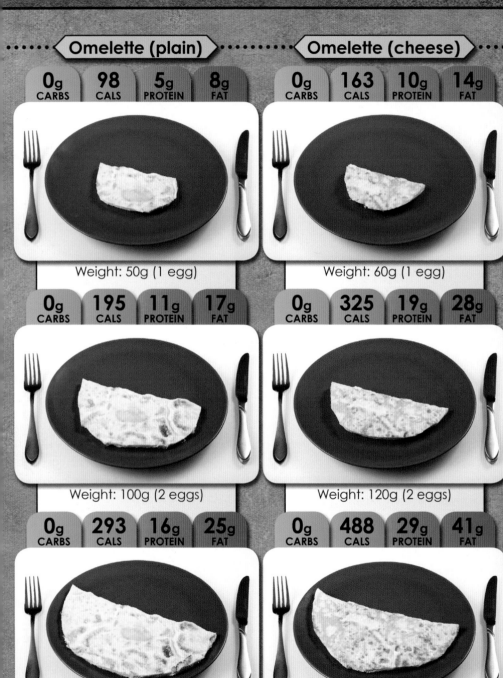

Omelette (plain)

| 0g CARBS | 98 CALS | 5g PROTEIN | 8g FAT |

Weight: 50g (1 egg)

| 0g CARBS | 195 CALS | 11g PROTEIN | 17g FAT |

Weight: 100g (2 eggs)

| 0g CARBS | 293 CALS | 16g PROTEIN | 25g FAT |

Weight: 150g (3 eggs)

Omelette (cheese)

| 0g CARBS | 163 CALS | 10g PROTEIN | 14g FAT |

Weight: 60g (1 egg)

| 0g CARBS | 325 CALS | 19g PROTEIN | 28g FAT |

Weight: 120g (2 eggs)

| 0g CARBS | 488 CALS | 29g PROTEIN | 41g FAT |

Weight: 180g (3 eggs)

Blue Stilton

0g CARBS	144 CALS	8g PROTEIN	12g FAT

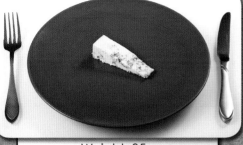

Weight: 35g

0g CARBS	287 CALS	17g PROTEIN	25g FAT

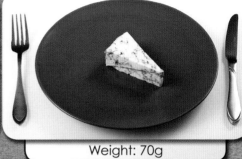

Weight: 70g

Brie

0g CARBS	86 CALS	5g PROTEIN	7g FAT

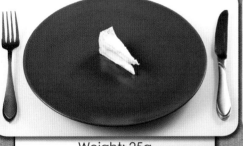

Weight: 25g

0g CARBS	172 CALS	10g PROTEIN	15g FAT

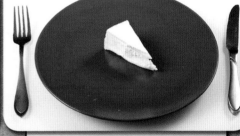

Weight: 50g

Camembert

0g CARBS	102 CALS	8g PROTEIN	8g FAT

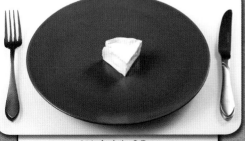

Weight: 35g

0g CARBS	203 CALS	15g PROTEIN	16g FAT

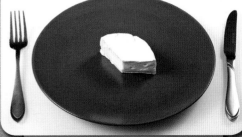

Weight: 70g

Cheddar

| 0g CARBS | 104 CALS | 6g PROTEIN | 9g FAT | | 0g CARBS | 208 CALS | 13g PROTEIN | 17g FAT |

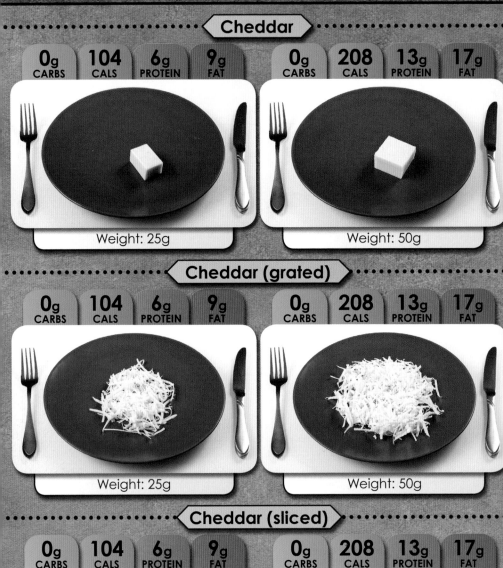

Weight: 25g   Weight: 50g

Cheddar (grated)

| 0g CARBS | 104 CALS | 6g PROTEIN | 9g FAT | | 0g CARBS | 208 CALS | 13g PROTEIN | 17g FAT |

Weight: 25g   Weight: 50g

Cheddar (sliced)

| 0g CARBS | 104 CALS | 6g PROTEIN | 9g FAT | | 0g CARBS | 208 CALS | 13g PROTEIN | 17g FAT |

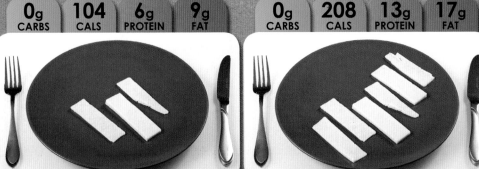

Weight: 25g   Weight: 50g

Cottage Cheese (plain)

2g CARBS	51 CALS	6g PROTEIN	2g FAT

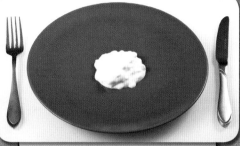

Weight: 50g

3g CARBS	101 CALS	13g PROTEIN	4g FAT

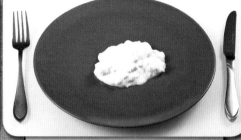

Weight: 100g

Edam

0g CARBS	85 CALS	7g PROTEIN	7g FAT

Weight: 25g

0g CARBS	171 CALS	13g PROTEIN	13g FAT

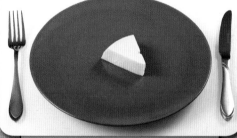

Weight: 50g

Feta

0g CARBS	75 CALS	5g PROTEIN	6g FAT

Weight: 30g

1g CARBS	150 CALS	9g PROTEIN	12g FAT

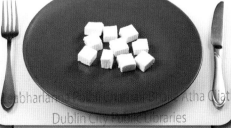

Weight: 60g

Goat's Cheese

0g CARBS	80 CALS	5g PROTEIN	6g FAT

1g CARBS	160 CALS	11g PROTEIN	13g FAT

Weight: 25g

Weight: 50g

Mozzarella

0g CARBS	64 CALS	5g PROTEIN	5g FAT

0g CARBS	129 CALS	9g PROTEIN	10g FAT

Weight: 25g

Weight: 50g

Parmesan

0g CARBS	42 CALS	4g PROTEIN	3g FAT

0g CARBS	83 CALS	7g PROTEIN	6g FAT

Weight: 10g

Weight: 20g

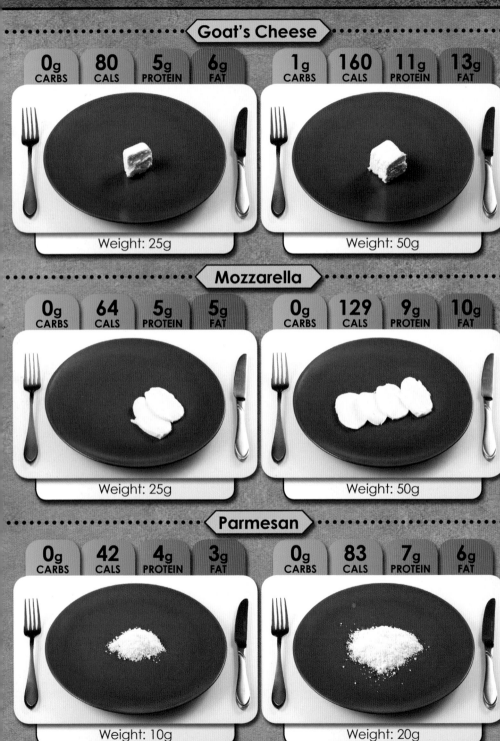

Red Leicester

0g CARBS	100 CALS	6g PROTEIN	8g FAT		0g CARBS	201 CALS	12g PROTEIN	17g FAT

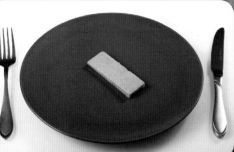

Weight: 25g

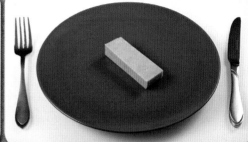

Weight: 50g

Processed Cheese Slice

1g CARBS	59 CALS	4g PROTEIN	5g FAT

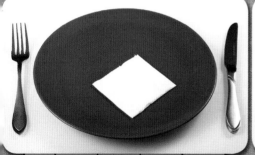

	CARBS	CALS	PROT	FAT
2x	2g	118	8g	10g
3x	3g	177	12g	15g
4x	4g	236	16g	20g

Weight: 20g

Spreadable Cheese

1g CARBS	48 CALS	2g PROTEIN	4g FAT

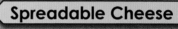

	CARBS	CALS	PROT	FAT
2x	2g	96	4g	8g
3x	3g	144	6g	12g
4x	4g	192	8g	16g

Weight: 18g

Soft Cheese

0g CARBS	94 CALS	2g PROTEIN	9g FAT

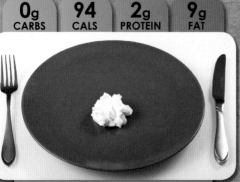

Weight: 30g

0g CARBS	187 CALS	5g PROTEIN	19g FAT

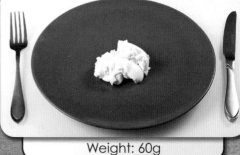

Weight: 60g

Squirty Cheese

0g CARBS	24 CALS	1g PROTEIN	2g FAT

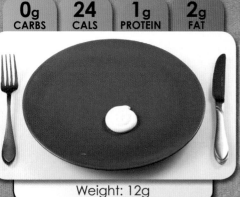

Weight: 12g

1g CARBS	48 CALS	3g PROTEIN	4g FAT

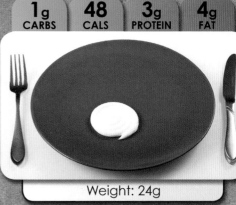

Weight: 24g

Wensleydale with Cranberries

2g CARBS	90 CALS	5g PROTEIN	7g FAT

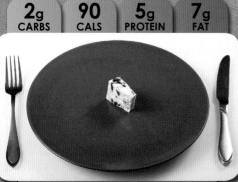

Weight: 25g

3g CARBS	180 CALS	10g PROTEIN	14g FAT

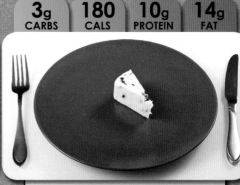

Weight: 50g

Apricot (fresh)

4g CARBS	17 CALS	0g PROTEIN	0g FAT

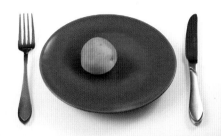

Weight: 55g

8g CARBS	34 CALS	1g PROTEIN	0g FAT

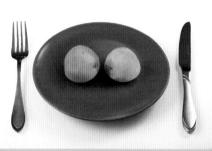

Weight: 110g

12g CARBS	51 CALS	1g PROTEIN	0g FAT

Weight: 165g

Apricot (dried)

10g CARBS	44 CALS	1g PROTEIN	0g FAT

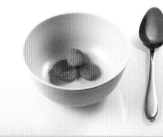

Weight: 28g

20g CARBS	87 CALS	2g PROTEIN	0g FAT

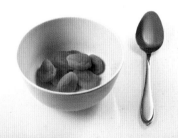

Weight: 55g

30g CARBS	130 CALS	3g PROTEIN	0g FAT

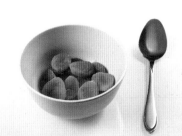

Weight: 82g

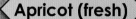

Apple

| 10g CARBS | 40 CALS | 0g PROTEIN | 0g FAT |

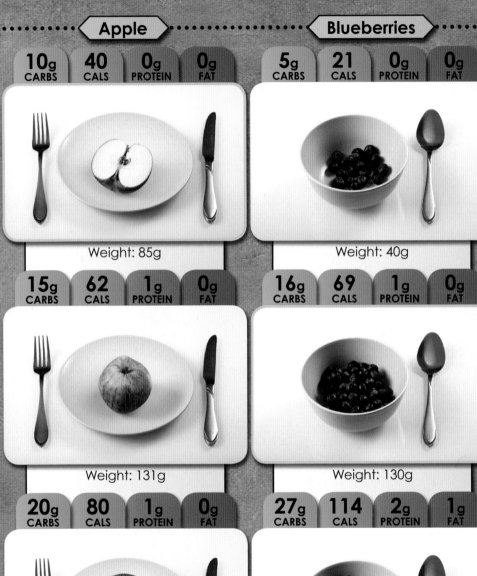

Weight: 85g

| 15g CARBS | 62 CALS | 1g PROTEIN | 0g FAT |

Weight: 131g

| 20g CARBS | 80 CALS | 1g PROTEIN | 0g FAT |

Weight: 170g

Blueberries

| 5g CARBS | 21 CALS | 0g PROTEIN | 0g FAT |

Weight: 40g

| 16g CARBS | 69 CALS | 1g PROTEIN | 0g FAT |

Weight: 130g

| 27g CARBS | 114 CALS | 2g PROTEIN | 1g FAT |

Weight: 215g

Banana

15g CARBS	60 CALS	1g PROTEIN	0g FAT

Weight: 63g (without skin)

15g CARBS	60 CALS	1g PROTEIN	0g FAT

Weight: 97g (with skin)

20g CARBS	81 CALS	1g PROTEIN	0g FAT

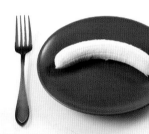

Weight: 85g (without skin)

20g CARBS	81 CALS	1g PROTEIN	0g FAT

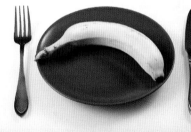

Weight: 130g (with skin)

30g CARBS	122 CALS	2g PROTEIN	0g FAT

Weight: 128g (without skin)

30g CARBS	122 CALS	2g PROTEIN	0g FAT

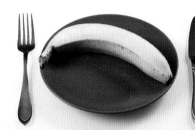

Weight: 190g (with skin)

Cherries

| 6g CARBS | 24 CALS | 0g PROTEIN | 0g FAT |

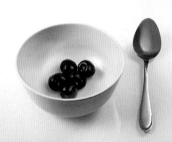

Weight: 50g (with stones)

| 12g CARBS | 48 CALS | 1g PROTEIN | 0g FAT |

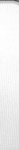

Weight: 100g (with stones)

| 18g CARBS | 77 CALS | 1g PROTEIN | 0g FAT |

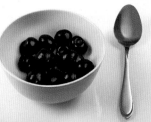

Weight: 160g (with stones)

Clementine

| 5g CARBS | 22 CALS | 1g PROTEIN | 0g FAT |

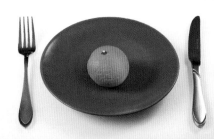

Weight: 80g

| 10g CARBS | 45 CALS | 1g PROTEIN | 0g FAT |

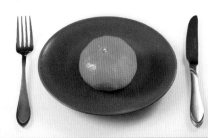

Weight: 160g

Satsuma

| 5g CARBS | 22 CALS | 1g PROTEIN | 0g FAT |

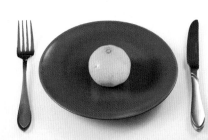

Weight: 85g

Fruit Cocktail (in juice)

5g CARBS	22 CALS	0g PROTEIN	0g FAT

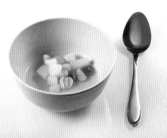

Weight: 75g

15g CARBS	61 CALS	1g PROTEIN	0g FAT

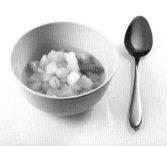

Weight: 210g (half tin)

30g CARBS	122 CALS	2g PROTEIN	0g FAT

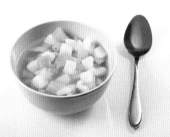

Weight: 420g (full tin)

Grapefruit

5g CARBS	24 CALS	1g PROTEIN	0g FAT

Weight: 119g (half)

10g CARBS	46 CALS	1g PROTEIN	0g FAT

Weight: 228g (whole)

10g CARBS	46 CALS	1g PROTEIN	0g FAT

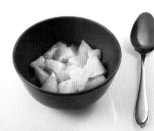

Weight: 140g (whole)

Grapes (seedless)

10g CARBS	39 CALS	0g PROTEIN	0g FAT

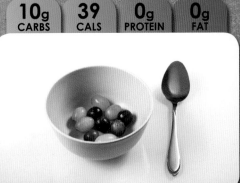

Weight: 65g

20g CARBS	78 CALS	1g PROTEIN	0g FAT

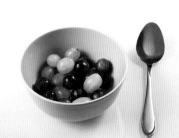

Weight: 130g

30g CARBS	117 CALS	1g PROTEIN	0g FAT

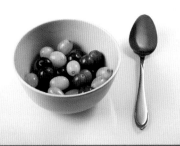

Weight: 195g

40g CARBS	156 CALS	1g PROTEIN	0g FAT

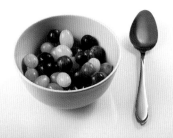

Weight: 260g

50g CARBS	195 CALS	1g PROTEIN	0g FAT

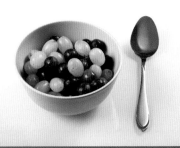

Weight: 325g

60g CARBS	234 CALS	2g PROTEIN	0g FAT

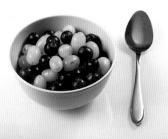

Weight: 390g

Kiwi

5g CARBS	24 CALS	1g PROTEIN	0g FAT

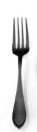
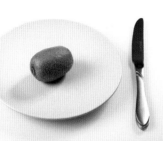
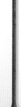

Weight: 55g (1 kiwi with skin)

5g CARBS	24 CALS	1g PROTEIN	0g FAT

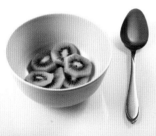
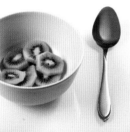
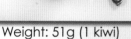

Weight: 51g (1 kiwi)

10g CARBS	47 CALS	1g PROTEIN	0g FAT

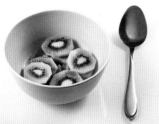
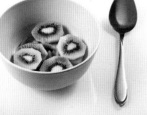
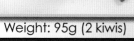

Weight: 95g (2 kiwis)

Mango

10g CARBS	40 CALS	0g PROTEIN	0g FAT

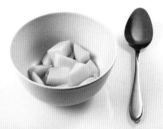
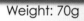

Weight: 70g

20g CARBS	80 CALS	1g PROTEIN	0g FAT

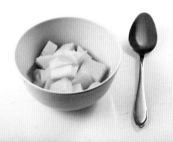

Weight: 140g

30g CARBS	120 CALS	1g PROTEIN	0g FAT

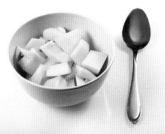

Weight: 210g

Melon (honeydew)   ## Watermelon

| **10**g CARBS | **42** CALS | **1**g PROTEIN | **0**g FAT | **10**g CARBS | **43** CALS | **1**g PROTEIN | **0**g FAT |

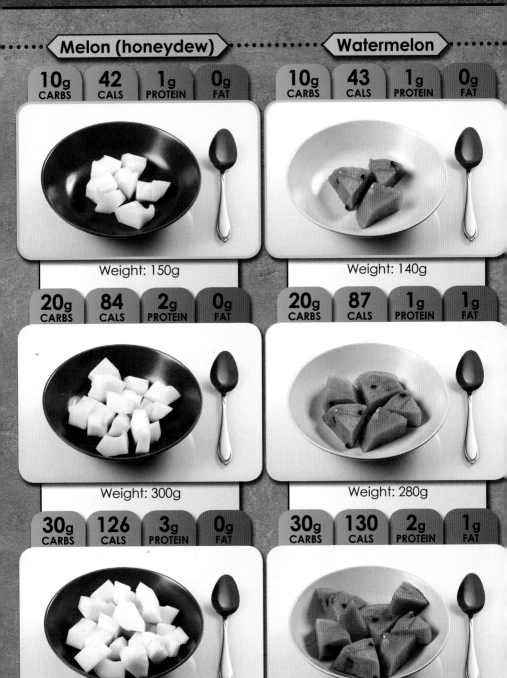

Weight: 150g

Weight: 140g

| **20**g CARBS | **84** CALS | **2**g PROTEIN | **0**g FAT | **20**g CARBS | **87** CALS | **1**g PROTEIN | **1**g FAT |

Weight: 300g

Weight: 280g

| **30**g CARBS | **126** CALS | **3**g PROTEIN | **0**g FAT | **30**g CARBS | **130** CALS | **2**g PROTEIN | **1**g FAT |

Weight: 450g

Weight: 420g

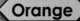 Orange

Papaya

4g CARBS	18 CALS	1g PROTEIN	0g FAT

5g CARBS	24 CALS	1g PROTEIN	0g FAT

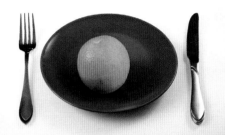

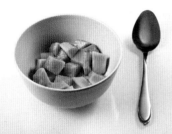

Weight: 71g

Weight: 90g

7g CARBS	30 CALS	1g PROTEIN	0g FAT

10g CARBS	49 CALS	2g PROTEIN	0g FAT

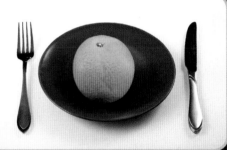

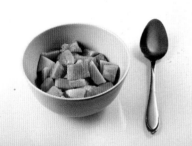

Weight: 115g

Weight: 180g

10g CARBS	45 CALS	1g PROTEIN	0g FAT

15g CARBS	73 CALS	2g PROTEIN	0g FAT

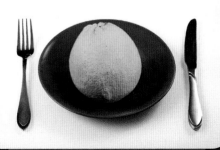

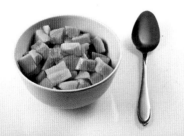

Weight: 172g

Weight: 270g

Peach (fresh)

5g CARBS	23 CALS	1g PROTEIN	0g FAT

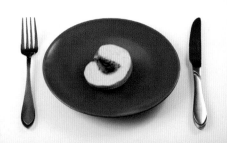

Weight: 70g (without stone)

10g CARBS	46 CALS	1g PROTEIN	0g FAT

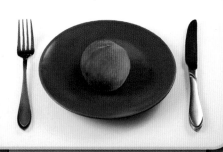

Weight: 138g

15g CARBS	66 CALS	2g PROTEIN	0g FAT

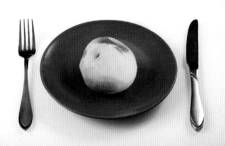

Weight: 200g

Peach (tinned in juice)

10g CARBS	39 CALS	1g PROTEIN	0g FAT

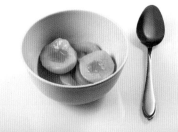

Weight: 100g

20g CARBS	80 CALS	1g PROTEIN	0g FAT

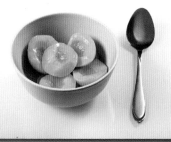

Weight: 205g (half tin)

40g CARBS	160 CALS	2g PROTEIN	0g FAT

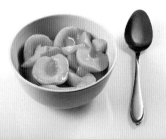

Weight: 410g (full tin)

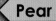 **Pear**

Pear (tinned in juice)

10g CARBS	42 CALS	0g PROTEIN	0g FAT

10g CARBS	38 CALS	0g PROTEIN	0g FAT

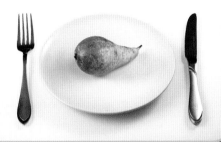

Weight: 104g

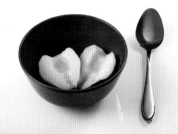

Weight: 115g

20g CARBS	78 CALS	1g PROTEIN	0g FAT

20g CARBS	76 CALS	1g PROTEIN	0g FAT

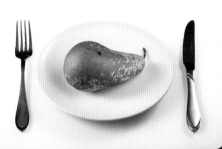

Weight: 195g

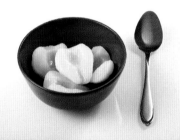

Weight: 230g

30g CARBS	118 CALS	1g PROTEIN	0g FAT

30g CARBS	117 CALS	1g PROTEIN	0g FAT

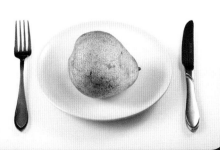

Weight: 295g

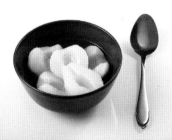

Weight: 355g (full tin)

Pineapple (fresh)

4g CARBS	16 CALS	0g PROTEIN	0g FAT

Weight: 40g

8g CARBS	33 CALS	0g PROTEIN	0g FAT

Weight: 80g

12g CARBS	49 CALS	0g PROTEIN	0g FAT

Weight: 120g

16g CARBS	66 CALS	1g PROTEIN	0g FAT

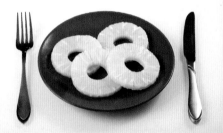

Weight: 160g

20g CARBS	82 CALS	1g PROTEIN	0g FAT

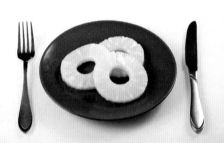

Weight: 200g

24g CARBS	98 CALS	1g PROTEIN	0g FAT

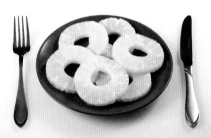

Weight: 240g

Pineapple (tinned in juice)

5g CARBS	**19** CALS	**0**g PROTEIN	**0**g FAT

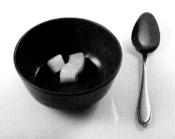

Weight: 40g

10g CARBS	**38** CALS	**0**g PROTEIN	**0**g FAT

Weight: 80g

20g CARBS	**75** CALS	**0**g PROTEIN	**0**g FAT

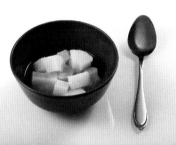

Weight: 160g

30g CARBS	**115** CALS	**1**g PROTEIN	**0**g FAT

Weight: 245g

40g CARBS	**155** CALS	**1**g PROTEIN	**0**g FAT

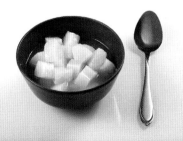

Weight: 330g

50g CARBS	**193** CALS	**1**g PROTEIN	**0**g FAT

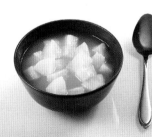

Weight: 410g (full tin)

Pomegranate

5g	20	1g	0g
CARBS	CALS	PROTEIN	FAT

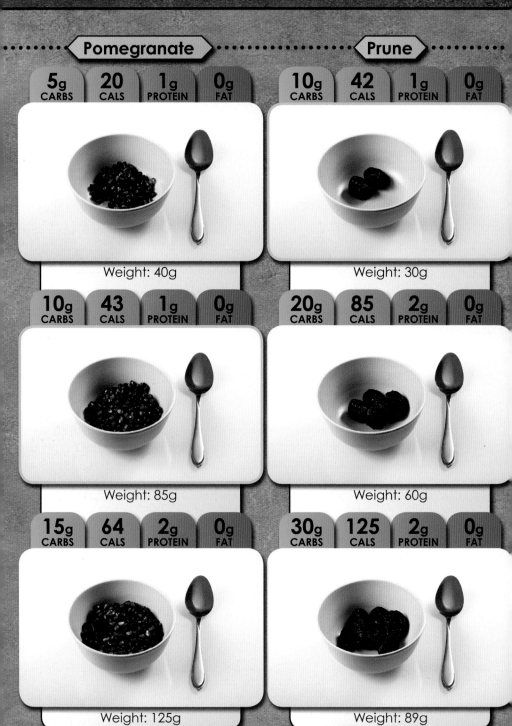

Weight: 40g

10g	43	1g	0g
CARBS	CALS	PROTEIN	FAT

Weight: 85g

15g	64	2g	0g
CARBS	CALS	PROTEIN	FAT

Weight: 125g

Prune

10g	42	1g	0g
CARBS	CALS	PROTEIN	FAT

Weight: 30g

20g	85	2g	0g
CARBS	CALS	PROTEIN	FAT

Weight: 60g

30g	125	2g	0g
CARBS	CALS	PROTEIN	FAT

Weight: 89g

Plum

| **5**g CARBS | **20** CALS | **0**g PROTEIN | **0**g FAT |

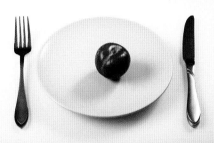

	CARBS	CALS	PROT	FAT
2x	10g	40	0g	0g
3x	15g	60	0g	0g
4x	20g	80	0g	0g
Weight: 55g				

| **10**g CARBS | **40** CALS | **1**g PROTEIN | **0**g FAT |

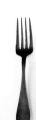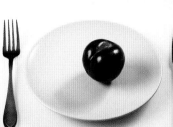

	CARBS	CALS	PROT	FAT
2x	20g	80	2g	0g
3x	30g	120	3g	0g
4x	40g	160	4g	0g
Weight: 110g				

Nectarine

| **7**g CARBS | **32** CALS | **1**g PROTEIN | **0**g FAT |

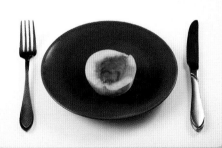

	CARBS	CALS	PROT	FAT
2x	14g	64	2g	0g
3x	21g	96	3g	0g
4x	28g	128	4g	0g
Weight: 80g (without stone)				

| **15**g CARBS | **66** CALS | **2**g PROTEIN | **0**g FAT |

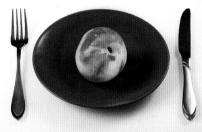

	CARBS	CALS	PROT	FAT
2x	30g	132	4g	0g
3x	45g	198	6g	0g
4x	60g	264	8g	0g
Weight: 165g				

Raspberries

| 5g CARBS | 26 CALS | 1g PROTEIN | 0g FAT |

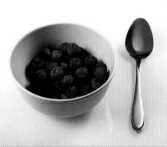

Weight: 105g

| 10g CARBS | 53 CALS | 3g PROTEIN | 1g FAT |

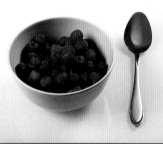

Weight: 210g

| 15g CARBS | 80 CALS | 4g PROTEIN | 1g FAT |

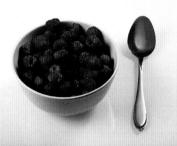

Weight: 320g

Strawberries

| 5g CARBS | 23 CALS | 1g PROTEIN | 0g FAT |

Weight: 85g

| 15g CARBS | 68 CALS | 2g PROTEIN | 0g FAT |

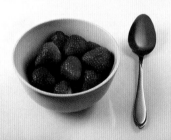

Weight: 250g

| 25g CARBS | 111 CALS | 3g PROTEIN | 0g FAT |

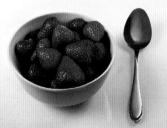

Weight: 410g

Raisins

| 10g CARBS | 41 CALS | 0g PROTEIN | 0g FAT |

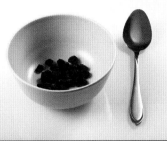

Weight: 15g

| 20g CARBS | 79 CALS | 1g PROTEIN | 0g FAT |

Weight: 29g

| 30g CARBS | 120 CALS | 1g PROTEIN | 0g FAT |

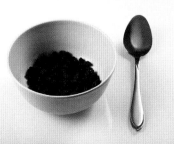

Weight: 44g

Sultanas

| 10g CARBS | 41 CALS | 0g PROTEIN | 0g FAT |

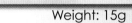

Weight: 15g

| 20g CARBS | 80 CALS | 1g PROTEIN | 0g FAT |

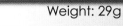

Weight: 29g

| 30g CARBS | 118 CALS | 1g PROTEIN | 0g FAT |

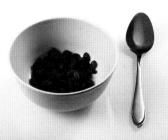

Weight: 43g

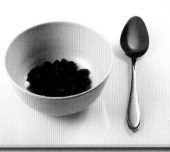

Beans on Toast (with margarine)

22g CARBS	151 CALS	5g PROTEIN	4g FAT

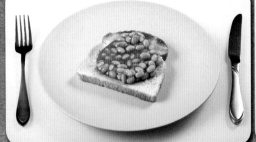

22g toast, 65g beans, 5g marg

32g CARBS	205 CALS	9g PROTEIN	5g FAT

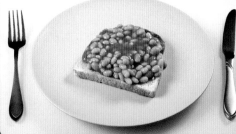

22g toast, 130g beans, 5g marg

42g CARBS	260 CALS	12g PROTEIN	5g FAT

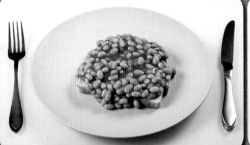

22g toast, 195g beans, 5g marg

55g CARBS	356 CALS	14g PROTEIN	10g FAT

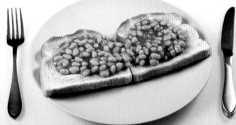

44g toast, 195g beans, 10g marg

70g CARBS	438 CALS	19g PROTEIN	11g FAT

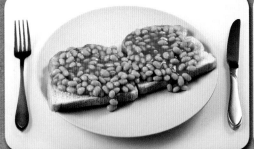

44g toast, 293g beans, 10g marg

85g CARBS	520 CALS	24g PROTEIN	11g FAT

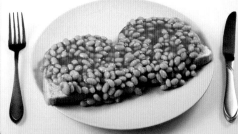

44g toast, 390g beans, 10g marg

Chicken Goujons, Potato Faces & Peas

18g CARBS	172 CALS	9g PROTEIN	9g FAT

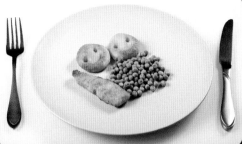

30g chick, 34g faces, 25g peas

38g CARBS	346 CALS	17g PROTEIN	19g FAT

60g chick, 68g faces, 50g peas

56g CARBS	518 CALS	25g PROTEIN	29g FAT

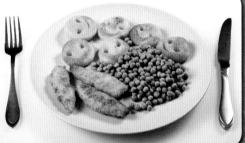

90g chick, 102g faces, 75g peas

76g CARBS	691 CALS	33g PROTEIN	38g FAT

120g chick, 136g faces, 100g peas

93g CARBS	864 CALS	42g PROTEIN	47g FAT

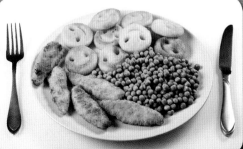

150g chick, 170g faces, 125g peas

113g CARBS	1038 CALS	50g PROTEIN	57g FAT

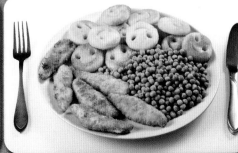

180g chick, 204g faces, 150g peas

Chilli con Carne with White Rice

15g CARBS	137 CALS	8g PROTEIN	5g FAT

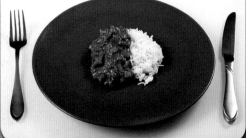

90g chilli, 32g rice

40g CARBS	307 CALS	15g PROTEIN	10g FAT

170g chilli, 96g rice

65g CARBS	483 CALS	23g PROTEIN	16g FAT

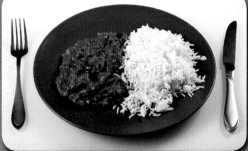

250g chilli, 163g rice

91g CARBS	661 CALS	32g PROTEIN	22g FAT

340g chilli, 225g rice

116g CARBS	843 CALS	41g PROTEIN	28g FAT

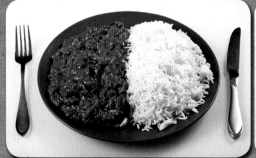

430g chilli, 290g rice

141g CARBS	1015 CALS	48g PROTEIN	33g FAT

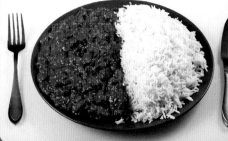

510g chilli, 355g rice

Corned Beef Hash

12g CARBS	141 CALS	11g PROTEIN	6g FAT

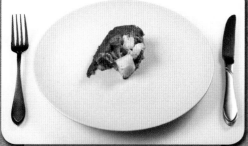

Weight: 100g

25g CARBS	282 CALS	21g PROTEIN	12g FAT

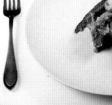

Weight: 200g

37g CARBS	423 CALS	32g PROTEIN	18g FAT

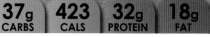

Weight: 300g

49g CARBS	564 CALS	42g PROTEIN	24g FAT

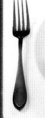
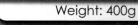

Weight: 400g

62g CARBS	705 CALS	53g PROTEIN	30g FAT

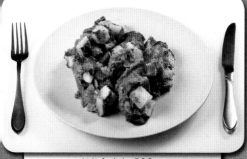

Weight: 500g

74g CARBS	846 CALS	63g PROTEIN	35g FAT

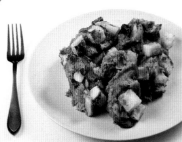

Weight: 600g

Curry (chicken) with White Rice

| **12g** CARBS | **146** CALS | **10g** PROTEIN | **3g** FAT |

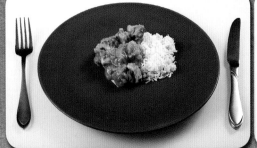

105g curry, 31g rice

| **35g** CARBS | **390** CALS | **26g** PROTEIN | **8g** FAT |

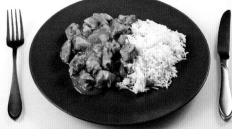

260g curry, 98g rice

| **57g** CARBS | **580** CALS | **36g** PROTEIN | **11g** FAT |

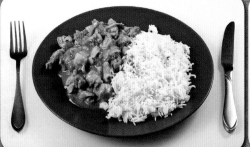

365g curry, 161g rice

| **79g** CARBS | **810** CALS | **50g** PROTEIN | **16g** FAT |

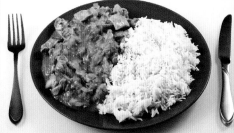

505g curry, 228g rice

| **101g** CARBS | **1013** CALS | **62g** PROTEIN | **20g** FAT |

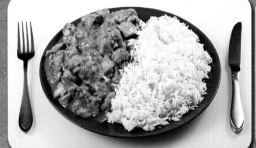

625g curry, 290g rice

| **124g** CARBS | **1267** CALS | **78g** PROTEIN | **25g** FAT |

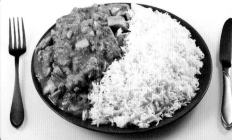

790g curry, 357g rice

Curry (lentil) with Brown Rice

20g CARBS	179 CALS	5g PROTEIN	9g FAT

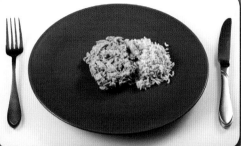

95g curry, 30g rice

49g CARBS	400 CALS	11g PROTEIN	19g FAT

185g curry, 95g rice

79g CARBS	624 CALS	17g PROTEIN	29g FAT

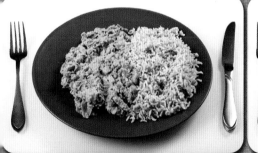

280g curry, 157g rice

110g CARBS	856 CALS	23g PROTEIN	38g FAT

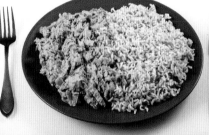

380g curry, 219g rice

140g CARBS	1080 CALS	29g PROTEIN	49g FAT

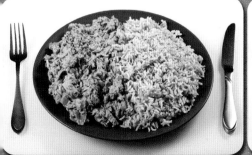

475g curry, 281g rice

170g CARBS	1306 CALS	35g PROTEIN	59g FAT

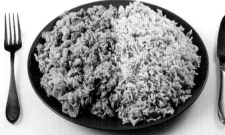

570g curry, 344g rice

Curry (veg & potato) with White Rice

20g CARBS	120 CALS	3g PROTEIN	4g FAT

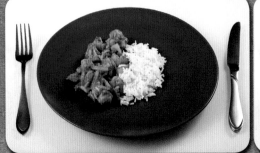

90g curry, 32g rice

49g CARBS	281 CALS	7g PROTEIN	8g FAT

175g curry, 97g rice

78g CARBS	443 CALS	9g PROTEIN	12g FAT

260g curry, 163g rice

108g CARBS	607 CALS	13g PROTEIN	17g FAT

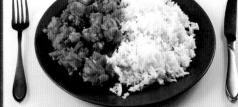

350g curry, 227g rice

138g CARBS	772 CALS	17g PROTEIN	21g FAT

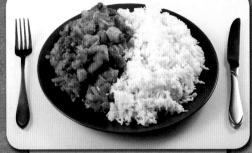

440g curry, 291g rice

167g CARBS	935 CALS	20g PROTEIN	26g FAT

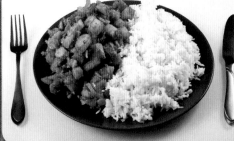

530g curry, 355g rice

Fish Fingers (grilled), Chips (oven) & Beans

30g CARBS	185 CALS	7g PROTEIN	5g FAT

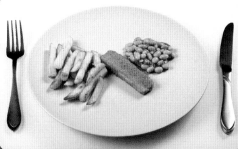

20g fish, 66g chips, 45g beans

51g CARBS	316 CALS	14g PROTEIN	9g FAT

40g fish, 99g chips, 90g beans

70g CARBS	444 CALS	20g PROTEIN	11g FAT

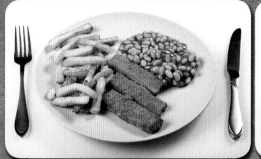

60g fish, 130g chips, 135g beans

90g CARBS	578 CALS	25g PROTEIN	15g FAT

80g fish, 165g chips, 180g beans

111g CARBS	714 CALS	32g PROTEIN	18g FAT

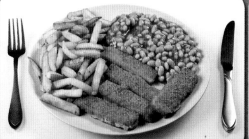

100g fish, 198g chips, 230g beans

131g CARBS	844 CALS	38g PROTEIN	23g FAT

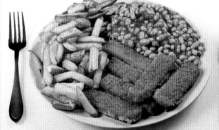

120g fish, 230g chips, 275g beans

Fish Pie

| 11g CARBS | 148 CALS | 11g PROTEIN | 7g FAT |

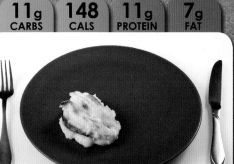

Weight: 125g

| 22g CARBS | 295 CALS | 22g PROTEIN | 14g FAT |

Weight: 250g

| 34g CARBS | 448 CALS | 34g PROTEIN | 21g FAT |

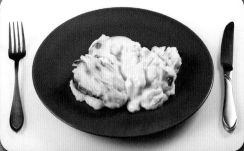

Weight: 380g

| 45g CARBS | 596 CALS | 45g PROTEIN | 27g FAT |

Weight: 505g

| 56g CARBS | 743 CALS | 56g PROTEIN | 34g FAT |

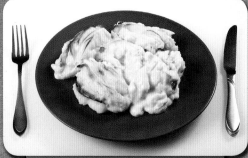

Weight: 630g

| 68g CARBS | 897 CALS | 68g PROTEIN | 41g FAT |

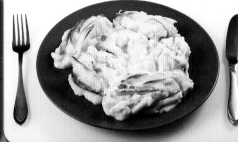

Weight: 760g

Lasagne

10g CARBS	146 CALS	8g PROTEIN	8g FAT

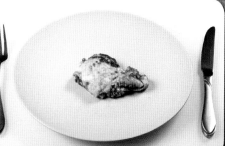

Weight: 80g

25g CARBS	357 CALS	20g PROTEIN	20g FAT

Weight: 195g

40g CARBS	576 CALS	33g PROTEIN	33g FAT

Weight: 315g

55g CARBS	787 CALS	45g PROTEIN	45g FAT

Weight: 430g

70g CARBS	997 CALS	57g PROTEIN	57g FAT

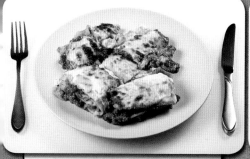

Weight: 545g

85g CARBS	1217 CALS	70g PROTEIN	69g FAT

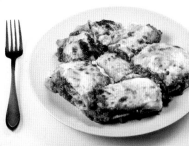

Weight: 665g

Macaroni Cheese

14g CARBS	**166** CALS	**7g** PROTEIN	**9g** FAT

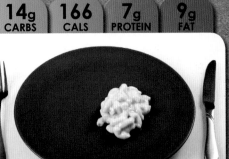

Weight: 80g

30g CARBS	**337** CALS	**15g** PROTEIN	**18g** FAT

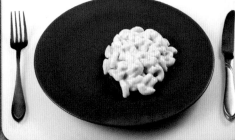

Weight: 163g

40g CARBS	**460** CALS	**20g** PROTEIN	**25g** FAT

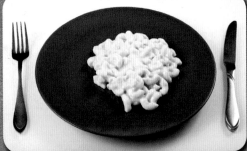

Weight: 222g

55g CARBS	**629** CALS	**28g** PROTEIN	**34g** FAT

Weight: 304g

70g CARBS	**797** CALS	**35g** PROTEIN	**43g** FAT

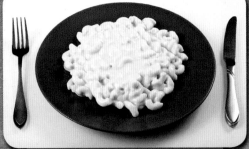

Weight: 385g

84g CARBS	**963** CALS	**42g** PROTEIN	**52g** FAT

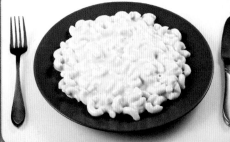

Weight: 465g

Enchilada (chicken)

	CARBS	CALS	PROT	FAT
29g CARBS	**323** CALS	**24g** PROTEIN	**14g** FAT	

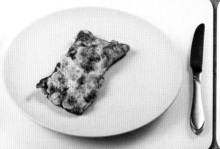

	CARBS	CALS	PROT	FAT
2x	58g	646	48g	28g
3x	87g	969	72g	42g
4x	116g	1292	96g	56g

Weight: 146g

Fajita (chicken)

30g CARBS	**245** CALS	**18g** PROTEIN	**5g** FAT

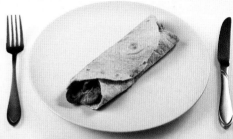

	CARBS	CALS	PROT	FAT
2x	60g	490	36g	10g
3x	90g	735	54g	15g
4x	120g	980	72g	20g

Weight: 160g

Quesadilla (bean)

19g CARBS	**166** CALS	**6g** PROTEIN	**7g** FAT

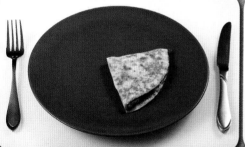

	CARBS	CALS	PROT	FAT
2x	38g	332	12g	14g
3x	57g	498	18g	21g
4x	76g	664	24g	28g

Weight: 74g

Taco (beef)

10g CARBS	**238** CALS	**12g** PROTEIN	**16g** FAT

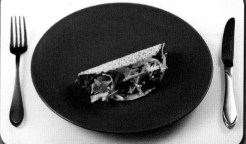

	CARBS	CALS	PROT	FAT
2x	20g	476	24g	32g
3x	30g	714	36g	48g
4x	40g	952	48g	64g

Weight: 80g

Pasta Bake (tuna & cheese)

15g CARBS	109 CALS	6g PROTEIN	3g FAT

Weight: 70g

30g CARBS	223 CALS	12g PROTEIN	6g FAT

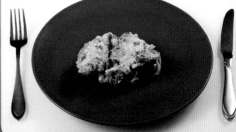

Weight: 143g

45g CARBS	334 CALS	18g PROTEIN	9g FAT

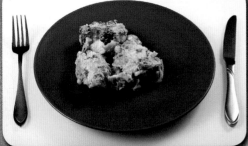

Weight: 214g

60g CARBS	439 CALS	23g PROTEIN	13g FAT

Weight: 285g

75g CARBS	547 CALS	29g PROTEIN	16g FAT

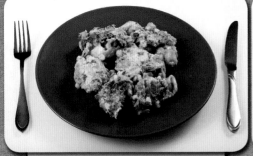

Weight: 355g

90g CARBS	665 CALS	35g PROTEIN	19g FAT

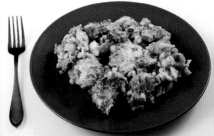

Weight: 426g

Pasta Meal (chicken & broccoli)

10g CARBS	110 CALS	5g PROTEIN	6g FAT

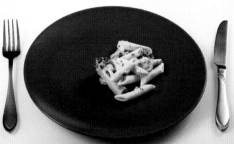

Weight: 65g

25g CARBS	281 CALS	13g PROTEIN	14g FAT

Weight: 166g

40g CARBS	451 CALS	21g PROTEIN	23g FAT

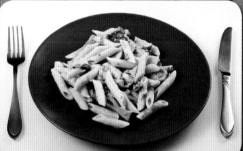

Weight: 267g

51g CARBS	576 CALS	27g PROTEIN	29g FAT

Weight: 341g

67g CARBS	747 CALS	34g PROTEIN	38g FAT

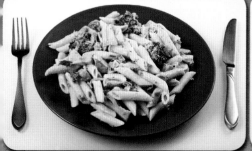

Weight: 442g

82g CARBS	918 CALS	42g PROTEIN	46g FAT

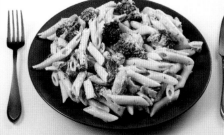

Weight: 543g

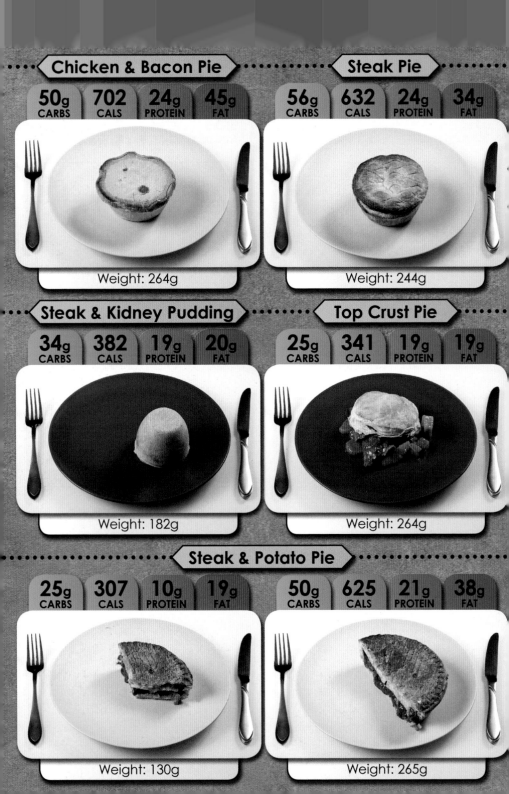

Chicken & Bacon Pie

| 50g CARBS | 702 CALS | 24g PROTEIN | 45g FAT |

Weight: 264g

Steak Pie

| 56g CARBS | 632 CALS | 24g PROTEIN | 34g FAT |

Weight: 244g

Steak & Kidney Pudding

| 34g CARBS | 382 CALS | 19g PROTEIN | 20g FAT |

Weight: 182g

Top Crust Pie

| 25g CARBS | 341 CALS | 19g PROTEIN | 19g FAT |

Weight: 264g

Steak & Potato Pie

| 25g CARBS | 307 CALS | 10g PROTEIN | 19g FAT |

Weight: 130g

| 50g CARBS | 625 CALS | 21g PROTEIN | 38g FAT |

Weight: 265g

Pizza (chicken, deep pan, oven baked)

20g CARBS	**143** CALS	**6g** PROTEIN	**4g** FAT

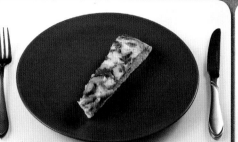

	CARBS	CALS	PROT	FAT
2x	40g	286	12g	8g
3x	60g	429	18g	12g
4x	80g	572	24g	16g
Weight: 65g				

40g CARBS	**286** CALS	**13g** PROTEIN	**8g** FAT

	CARBS	CALS	PROT	FAT
2x	80g	572	26g	16g
3x	120g	858	39g	24g
4x	160g	1144	52g	32g
Weight: 130g				

61g CARBS	**429** CALS	**19g** PROTEIN	**12g** FAT

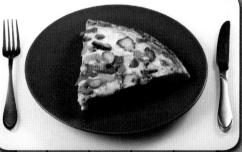

	CARBS	CALS	PROT	FAT
2x	122g	858	38g	24g
3x	183g	1287	57g	36g
4x	244g	1716	76g	48g
Weight: 195g				

80g CARBS	**568** CALS	**26g** PROTEIN	**16g** FAT

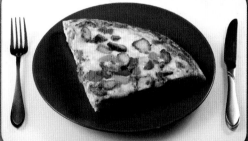

	CARBS	CALS	PROT	FAT
2x	160g	1136	52g	32g
3x	240g	1704	78g	48g
4x	320g	2272	104g	64g
Weight: 258g				

Pizza (pepperoni, thin crust, oven baked)

11g CARBS	102 CALS	5g PROTEIN	5g FAT

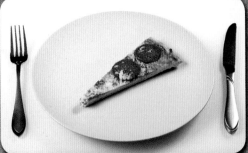

	CARBS	CALS	PROT	FAT
2x	22g	204	10g	10g
3x	33g	306	15g	15g
4x	44g	408	20g	20g
Weight: 40g				

20g CARBS	191 CALS	9g PROTEIN	8g FAT

	CARBS	CALS	PROT	FAT
2x	40g	382	18g	16g
3x	60g	573	27g	24g
4x	80g	764	36g	32g
Weight: 75g				

30g CARBS	293 CALS	14g PROTEIN	13g FAT

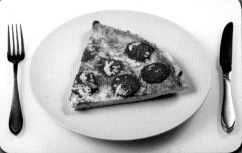

	CARBS	CALS	PROT	FAT
2x	60g	586	28g	26g
3x	90g	879	42g	39g
4x	120g	1172	56g	52g
Weight: 115g				

41g CARBS	395 CALS	20g PROTEIN	18g FAT

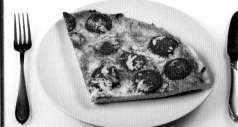

	CARBS	CALS	PROT	FAT
2x	82g	790	40g	36g
3x	123g	1185	60g	54g
4x	164g	1580	80g	72g
Weight: 155g				

Quiche Lorraine, Salad & Coleslaw

16g CARBS	410 CALS	11g PROTEIN	34g FAT

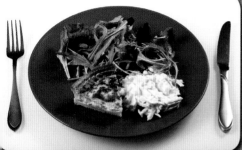

65g quiche, 65g coleslaw

29g CARBS	668 CALS	22g PROTEIN	52g FAT

135g quiche, 65g coleslaw

44g CARBS	1074 CALS	32g PROTEIN	86g FAT

200g quiche, 130g coleslaw

57g CARBS	1314 CALS	42g PROTEIN	103g FAT

265g quiche, 130g coleslaw

73g CARBS	1722 CALS	52g PROTEIN	137g FAT

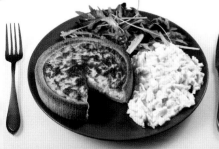

330g quiche, 195g coleslaw

86g CARBS	1980 CALS	63g PROTEIN	155g FAT

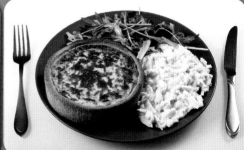

400g quiche, 195g coleslaw

Risotto (mushroom)

20g CARBS	169 CALS	5g PROTEIN	8g FAT

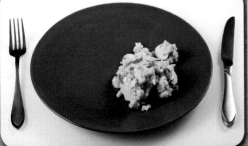

Weight: 120g

40g CARBS	340 CALS	9g PROTEIN	15g FAT

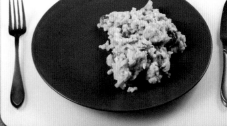

Weight: 241g

60g CARBS	512 CALS	14g PROTEIN	23g FAT

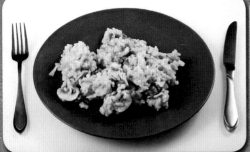

Weight: 363g

80g CARBS	684 CALS	19g PROTEIN	31g FAT

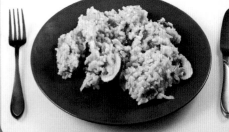

Weight: 485g

100g CARBS	856 CALS	24g PROTEIN	38g FAT

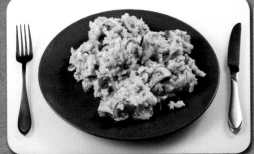

Weight: 607g

120g CARBS	1028 CALS	28g PROTEIN	46g FAT

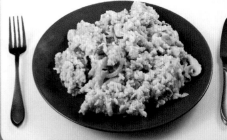

Weight: 729g

Sausage, Mash (with butter) & Onion Gravy ...

25g CARBS	297 CALS	10g PROTEIN	18g FAT

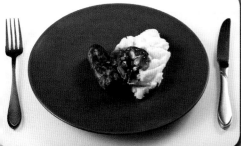

55g saus, 120g mash, 25g gravy

49g CARBS	587 CALS	21g PROTEIN	35g FAT

110g saus, 235g mash, 50g gravy

73g CARBS	883 CALS	31g PROTEIN	53g FAT

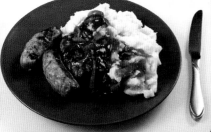

165g saus, 355g mash, 75g gravy

98g CARBS	1175 CALS	42g PROTEIN	71g FAT

220g saus, 470g mash, 100g gravy

122g CARBS	1472 CALS	53g PROTEIN	89g FAT

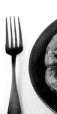

275g saus, 590g mash, 125g gravy

146g CARBS	1762 CALS	64g PROTEIN	106g FAT

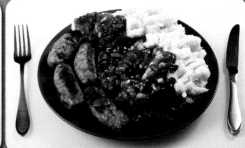

330g saus, 705g mash, 150g gravy

Shepherd's Pie

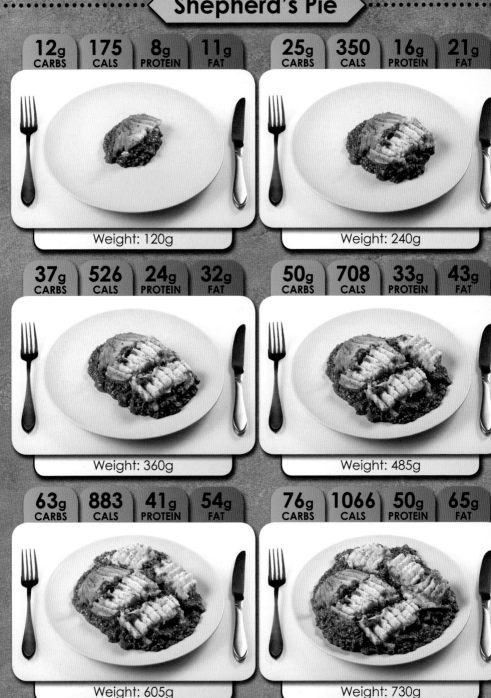

| 12g CARBS | 175 CALS | 8g PROTEIN | 11g FAT |

Weight: 120g

| 25g CARBS | 350 CALS | 16g PROTEIN | 21g FAT |

Weight: 240g

| 37g CARBS | 526 CALS | 24g PROTEIN | 32g FAT |

Weight: 360g

| 50g CARBS | 708 CALS | 33g PROTEIN | 43g FAT |

Weight: 485g

| 63g CARBS | 883 CALS | 41g PROTEIN | 54g FAT |

Weight: 605g

| 76g CARBS | 1066 CALS | 50g PROTEIN | 65g FAT |

Weight: 730g

Chicken Noodle Soup

4g CARBS	**25** CALS	**1**g PROTEIN	**0**g FAT

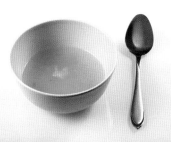

Weight: 130g

8g CARBS	**49** CALS	**3**g PROTEIN	**1**g FAT

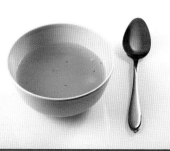

Weight: 260g

13g CARBS	**76** CALS	**4**g PROTEIN	**1**g FAT

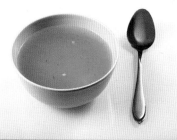

Weight: 400g

Chunky Veg Soup

13g CARBS	**64** CALS	**2**g PROTEIN	**1**g FAT

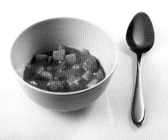

Weight: 133g

26g CARBS	**128** CALS	**4**g PROTEIN	**2**g FAT

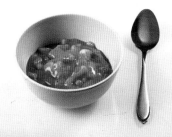

Weight: 266g

40g CARBS	**192** CALS	**6**g PROTEIN	**2**g FAT

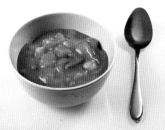

Weight: 400g

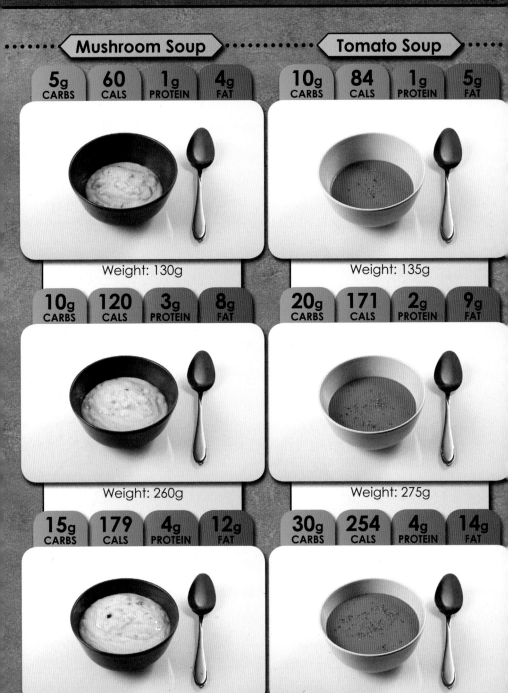

Mushroom Soup

| 5g CARBS | 60 CALS | 1g PROTEIN | 4g FAT |

Weight: 130g

| 10g CARBS | 120 CALS | 3g PROTEIN | 8g FAT |

Weight: 260g

| 15g CARBS | 179 CALS | 4g PROTEIN | 12g FAT |

Weight: 390g

Tomato Soup

| 10g CARBS | 84 CALS | 1g PROTEIN | 5g FAT |

Weight: 135g

| 20g CARBS | 171 CALS | 2g PROTEIN | 9g FAT |

Weight: 275g

| 30g CARBS | 254 CALS | 4g PROTEIN | 14g FAT |

Weight: 410g

Spaghetti Bolognaise

15g CARBS	144 CALS	9g PROTEIN	5g FAT

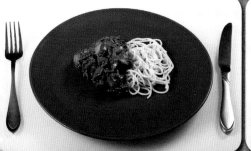

33g spag, 120g bolognaise

40g CARBS	334 CALS	18g PROTEIN	11g FAT

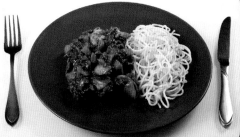

95g spag, 240g bolognaise

65g CARBS	527 CALS	28g PROTEIN	17g FAT

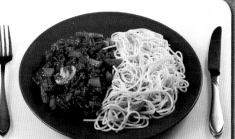

159g spag, 360g bolognaise

90g CARBS	720 CALS	39g PROTEIN	23g FAT

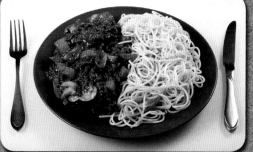

223g spag, 480g bolognaise

115g CARBS	915 CALS	49g PROTEIN	29g FAT

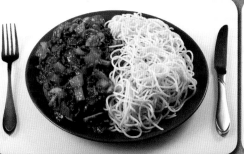

286g spag, 605g bolognaise

140g CARBS	1114 CALS	59g PROTEIN	35g FAT

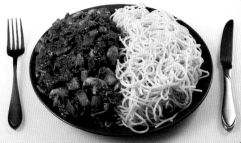

349g spag, 735g bolognaise

Stew & Dumplings

20g CARBS	**204** CALS	**9**g PROTEIN	**10**g FAT

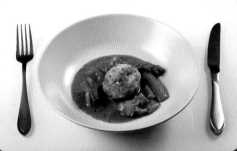

95g stew, 45g dumplings

40g CARBS	**397** CALS	**17**g PROTEIN	**20**g FAT

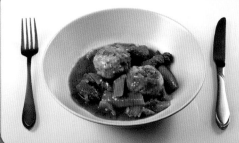

175g stew, 90g dumplings

65g CARBS	**658** CALS	**33**g PROTEIN	**31**g FAT

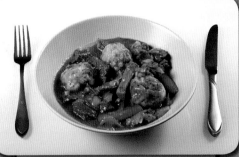

355g stew, 135g dumplings

85g CARBS	**855** CALS	**41**g PROTEIN	**41**g FAT

440g stew, 180g dumplings

105g CARBS	**1062** CALS	**51**g PROTEIN	**51**g FAT

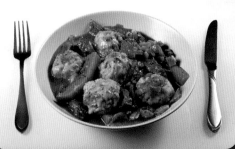

540g stew, 225g dumplings

125g CARBS	**1259** CALS	**60**g PROTEIN	**61**g FAT

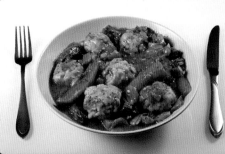

625g stew, 270g dumplings

Stir-fry (chicken)

10g CARBS	81 CALS	8g PROTEIN	2g FAT

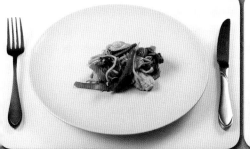

Weight: 70g

21g CARBS	162 CALS	15g PROTEIN	4g FAT

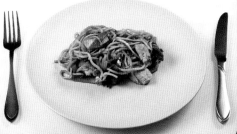

Weight: 140g

30g CARBS	238 CALS	22g PROTEIN	5g FAT

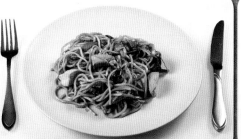

Weight: 205g

41g CARBS	319 CALS	30g PROTEIN	7g FAT

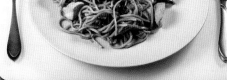

Weight: 275g

51g CARBS	400 CALS	37g PROTEIN	9g FAT

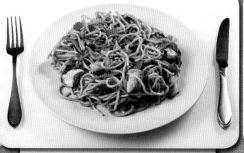

Weight: 345g

61g CARBS	477 CALS	44g PROTEIN	10g FAT

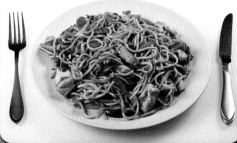

Weight: 411g

Sushi

9g CARBS	**53** CALS	**2g** PROTEIN	**1g** FAT

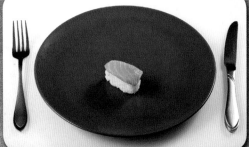

	CARBS	CALS	PROT	FAT
2x	18g	106	4g	2g
3x	27g	159	6g	3g
4x	36g	212	8g	4g
Weight: 34g				

10g CARBS	**58** CALS	**2g** PROTEIN	**1g** FAT

	CARBS	CALS	PROT	FAT
2x	20g	116	4g	2g
3x	30g	174	6g	3g
4x	40g	232	8g	4g
Weight: 36g				

8g CARBS	**44** CALS	**2g** PROTEIN	**1g** FAT

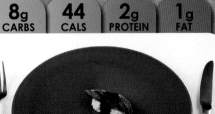
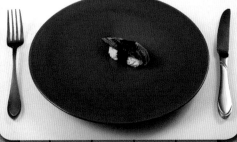

	CARBS	CALS	PROT	FAT
2x	16g	88	4g	2g
3x	24g	132	6g	3g
4x	32g	176	8g	4g
Weight: 28g				

6g CARBS	**40** CALS	**1g** PROTEIN	**1g** FAT

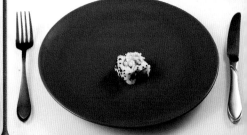

	CARBS	CALS	PROT	FAT
2x	12g	80	2g	2g
3x	18g	120	3g	3g
4x	24g	160	4g	4g
Weight: 24g				

Toad in the Hole

20g CARBS	269 CALS	12g PROTEIN	16g FAT

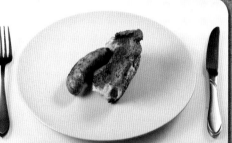

55g sausage, 37g yorkshire

40g CARBS	534 CALS	24g PROTEIN	32g FAT

110g sausage, 73g yorkshire

60g CARBS	803 CALS	37g PROTEIN	48g FAT

165g sausage, 110g yorkshire

80g CARBS	1069 CALS	49g PROTEIN	65g FAT

220g sausage, 146g yorkshire

100g CARBS	1335 CALS	61g PROTEIN	81g FAT

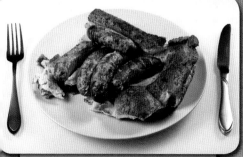

275g sausage, 182g yorkshire

119g CARBS	1603 CALS	73g PROTEIN	97g FAT

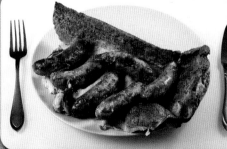

330g sausage, 219g yorkshire

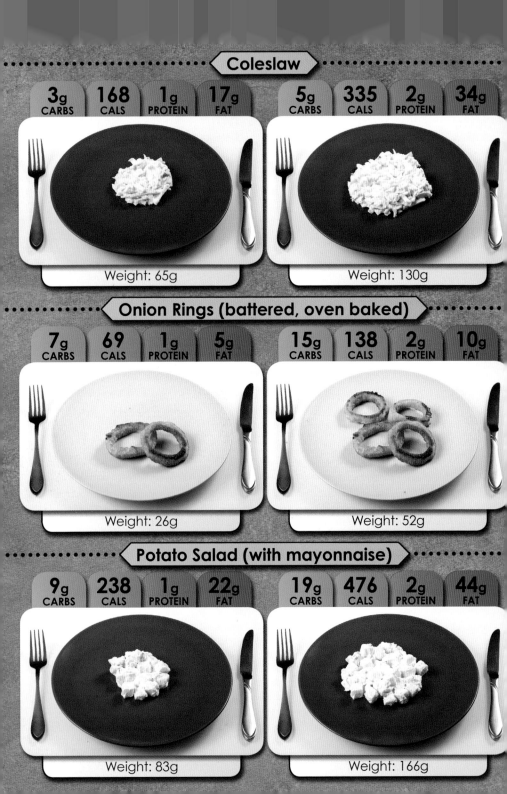

Coleslaw

3g CARBS	168 CALS	1g PROTEIN	17g FAT

Weight: 65g

5g CARBS	335 CALS	2g PROTEIN	34g FAT

Weight: 130g

Onion Rings (battered, oven baked)

7g CARBS	69 CALS	1g PROTEIN	5g FAT

Weight: 26g

15g CARBS	138 CALS	2g PROTEIN	10g FAT

Weight: 52g

Potato Salad (with mayonnaise)

9g CARBS	238 CALS	1g PROTEIN	22g FAT

Weight: 83g

19g CARBS	476 CALS	2g PROTEIN	44g FAT

Weight: 166g

Olives (pitted in brine)

0g CARBS	26 CALS	0g PROTEIN	3g FAT

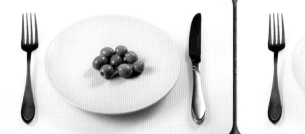

Weight: 25g

0g CARBS	52 CALS	0g PROTEIN	6g FAT

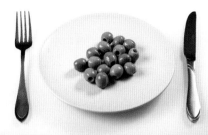

Weight: 50g

Pickled Onions

2g CARBS	8 CALS	0g PROTEIN	0g FAT

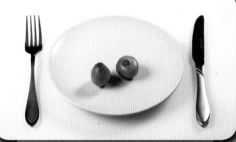

Weight: 35g

3g CARBS	17 CALS	1g PROTEIN	0g FAT

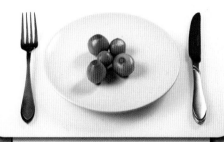

Weight: 70g

Sun-dried Tomatoes (in oil)

1g CARBS	124 CALS	1g PROTEIN	13g FAT

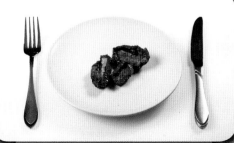

Weight: 25g

3g CARBS	248 CALS	2g PROTEIN	26g FAT

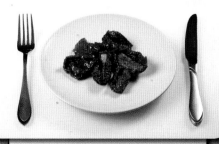

Weight: 50g

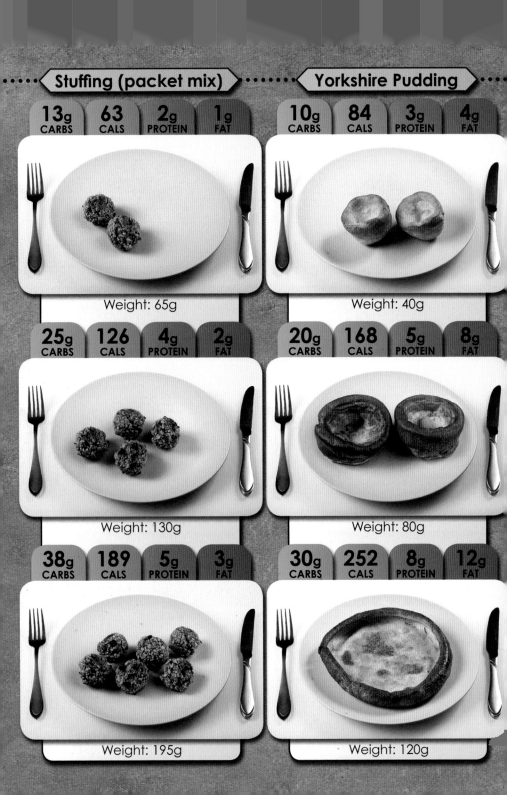

Stuffing (packet mix)

13g CARBS	63 CALS	2g PROTEIN	1g FAT

Weight: 65g

25g CARBS	126 CALS	4g PROTEIN	2g FAT

Weight: 130g

38g CARBS	189 CALS	5g PROTEIN	3g FAT

Weight: 195g

Yorkshire Pudding

10g CARBS	84 CALS	3g PROTEIN	4g FAT

Weight: 40g

20g CARBS	168 CALS	5g PROTEIN	8g FAT

Weight: 80g

30g CARBS	252 CALS	8g PROTEIN	12g FAT

Weight: 120g

Beef Burger (fried)

0g CARBS	329 CALS	29g PROTEIN	24g FAT

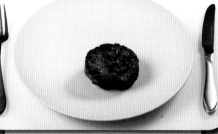

Weight: 100g

Corned Beef

0g CARBS	62 CALS	8g PROTEIN	3g FAT

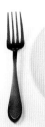

Weight: 30g

Sliced Beef

0g CARBS	69 CALS	13g PROTEIN	2g FAT

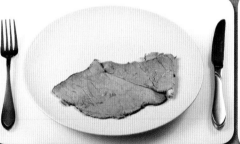

Weight: 50g

1g CARBS	127 CALS	16g PROTEIN	7g FAT

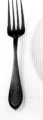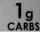

Weight: 62g

Wafer-thin Beef

0g CARBS	16 CALS	3g PROTEIN	0g FAT

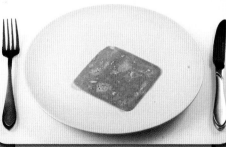

Weight: 12g

1g CARBS	189 CALS	24g PROTEIN	10g FAT

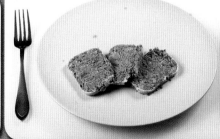

Weight: 92g

Rump Steak (fried)

0g CARBS	155 CALS	19g PROTEIN	9g FAT

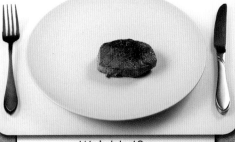

Weight: 68g

0g CARBS	442 CALS	55g PROTEIN	25g FAT

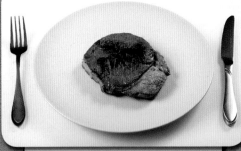

Weight: 194g

0g CARBS	951 CALS	118g PROTEIN	53g FAT

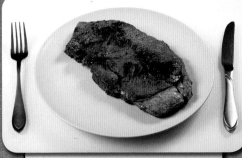

Weight: 417g

Sirloin Steak (fried)

0g CARBS	225 CALS	24g PROTEIN	14g FAT

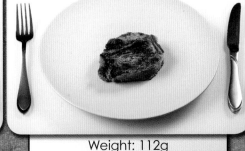

Weight: 112g

0g CARBS	394 CALS	42g PROTEIN	25g FAT

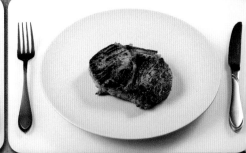

Weight: 196g

0g CARBS	527 CALS	57g PROTEIN	33g FAT

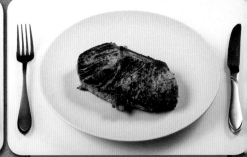

Weight: 262g

Roast Beef

0g CARBS	89 CALS	12g PROTEIN	5g FAT

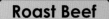

Weight: 40g

0g CARBS	167 CALS	22g PROTEIN	9g FAT

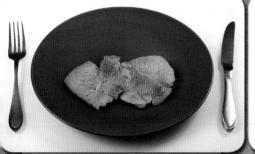

Weight: 75g

0g CARBS	278 CALS	37g PROTEIN	14g FAT

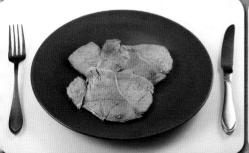

Weight: 125g

Roast Lamb

0g CARBS	96 CALS	11g PROTEIN	6g FAT

Weight: 40g

0g CARBS	180 CALS	21g PROTEIN	11g FAT

Weight: 75g

0g CARBS	300 CALS	35g PROTEIN	18g FAT

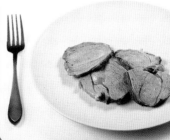

Weight: 125g

Lamb Chop (grilled)

0g CARBS	165 CALS	14g PROTEIN	12g FAT

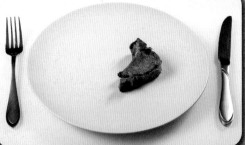

	CARBS	CALS	PROT	FAT
2x	0g	330	28g	24g
3x	0g	495	42g	36g
4x	0g	660	56g	48g
Weight: 54g				

0g CARBS	317 CALS	28g PROTEIN	23g FAT

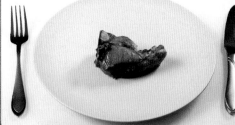

	CARBS	CALS	PROT	FAT
2x	0g	634	56g	46g
3x	0g	951	84g	69g
4x	0g	1268	112g	92g
Weight: 104g				

Lamb Steak (grilled)

0g CARBS	150 CALS	18g PROTEIN	9g FAT

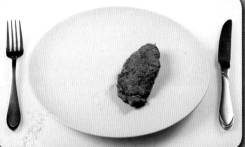

	CARBS	CALS	PROT	FAT
2x	0g	300	36g	18g
3x	0g	450	54g	27g
4x	0g	600	72g	36g
Weight: 65g				

0g CARBS	240 CALS	29g PROTEIN	14g FAT

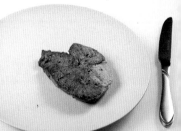

	CARBS	CALS	PROT	FAT
2x	0g	480	58g	28g
3x	0g	720	87g	42g
4x	0g	960	116g	56g
Weight: 104g				

Pork Chop (grilled)

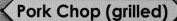

0g CARBS	175 CALS	20g PROTEIN	11g FAT

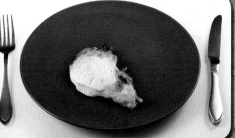

Weight: 68g

0g CARBS	514 CALS	58g PROTEIN	31g FAT

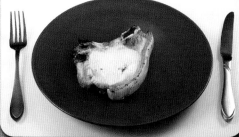

Weight: 200g

Gammon (grilled)

0g CARBS	169 CALS	24g PROTEIN	8g FAT

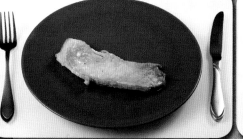

Weight: 85g

0g CARBS	338 CALS	48g PROTEIN	17g FAT

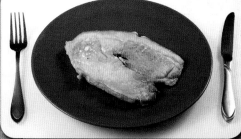

Weight: 170g

Roast Pork

0g CARBS	161 CALS	23g PROTEIN	8g FAT

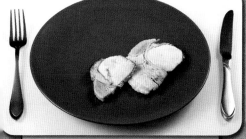

Weight: 75g

0g CARBS	269 CALS	39g PROTEIN	13g FAT

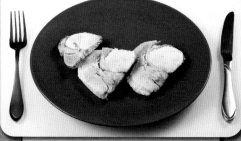

Weight: 125g

Back Bacon (fried)

| 0g CARBS | 74 CALS | 4g PROTEIN | 6g FAT |

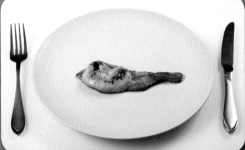

	CARBS	CALS	PROT	FAT
2x	0g	148	8g	12g
3x	0g	222	12g	18g
4x	0g	296	16g	24g
Weight: 16g

Back Bacon (grilled)

| 0g CARBS | 40 CALS | 3g PROTEIN | 3g FAT |

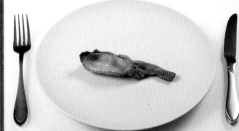

	CARBS	CALS	PROT	FAT
2x	0g	80	6g	6g
3x	0g	120	9g	9g
4x	0g	160	12g	12g
Weight: 14g

Streaky Bacon (fried)

| 0g CARBS | 54 CALS | 2g PROTEIN | 5g FAT |

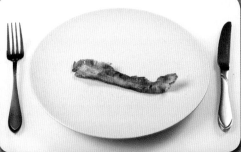

	CARBS	CALS	PROT	FAT
2x	0g	108	4g	10g
3x	0g	162	6g	15g
4x	0g	216	8g	20g
Weight: 11g

Streaky Bacon (grilled)

| 0g CARBS | 27 CALS | 2g PROTEIN | 2g FAT |

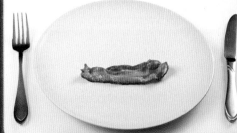

	CARBS	CALS	PROT	FAT
2x	0g	54	4g	4g
3x	0g	81	6g	6g
4x	0g	108	8g	8g
Weight: 8g

Chorizo

0g CARBS	17 CALS	1g PROTEIN	1g FAT

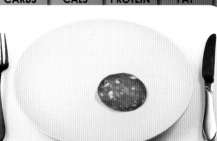

	CARBS	CALS	PROT	FAT
2x	0g	34	2g	2g
3x	0g	51	3g	3g
4x	0g	68	4g	4g
Weight: 6g				

Salami

0g CARBS	44 CALS	2g PROTEIN	4g FAT

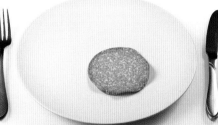

	CARBS	CALS	PROT	FAT
2x	0g	88	4g	8g
3x	0g	132	6g	12g
4x	0g	176	8g	16g
Weight: 10g				

Sliced Ham

0g CARBS	32 CALS	6g PROTEIN	1g FAT

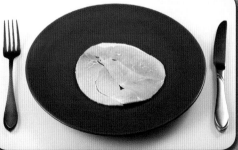

	CARBS	CALS	PROT	FAT
2x	0g	64	12g	2g
3x	0g	96	18g	3g
4x	0g	128	24g	4g
Weight: 30g				

Wafer-thin Ham

0g CARBS	13 CALS	2g PROTEIN	0g FAT

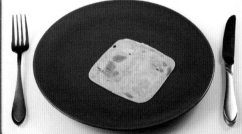

	CARBS	CALS	PROT	FAT
2x	0g	26	4g	0g
3x	0g	39	6g	0g
4x	0g	52	8g	0g
Weight: 12g				

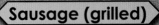

Sausage (grilled)

| 2g CARBS | 59 CALS | 3g PROTEIN | 4g FAT |

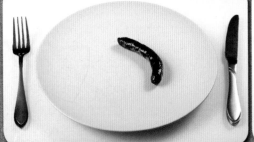

	CARBS	CALS	PROT	FAT
2x	4g	118	6g	8g
3x	6g	177	9g	12g
4x	8g	236	12g	16g
Weight: 20g (thin)				

| 5g CARBS | 162 CALS | 8g PROTEIN | 12g FAT |

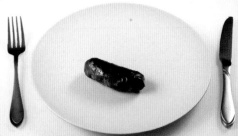

	CARBS	CALS	PROT	FAT
2x	10g	324	16g	24g
3x	15g	486	24g	36g
4x	20g	648	32g	48g
Weight: 55g (thick)				

Black Pudding (fried)

| 11g CARBS | 146 CALS | 6g PROTEIN | 9g FAT |

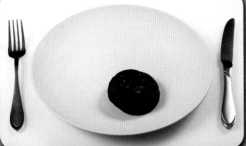

	CARBS	CALS	PROT	FAT
2x	22g	292	12g	18g
3x	33g	438	18g	27g
4x	44g	584	24g	36g
Weight: 58g				

Chicken Goujon (baked)

| 6g CARBS | 83 CALS | 6g PROTEIN | 4g FAT |

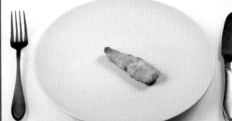

	CARBS	CALS	PROT	FAT
2x	12g	166	12g	8g
3x	18g	249	18g	12g
4x	24g	332	24g	16g
Weight: 30g				

Chicken Breast (skinless)

0g CARBS	**141** CALS	**30**g PROTEIN	**2**g FAT

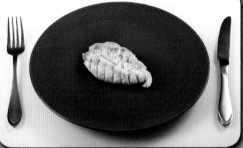

Weight: 95g (small)

0g CARBS	**296** CALS	**64**g PROTEIN	**4**g FAT

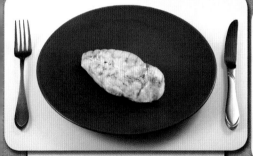

Weight: 200g (large)

Wafer-thin Chicken

1g CARBS	**16** CALS	**2**g PROTEIN	**1**g FAT

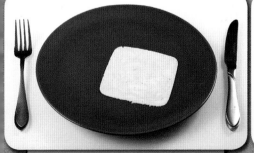

Weight: 12g

Roast Chicken (with skin)

0g CARBS	**163** CALS	**25**g PROTEIN	**7**g FAT

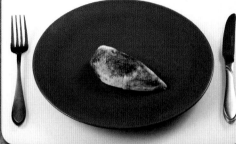

Weight: 92g

0g CARBS	**163** CALS	**25**g PROTEIN	**7**g FAT

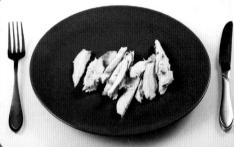

Weight: 92g

0g CARBS	**283** CALS	**44**g PROTEIN	**12**g FAT

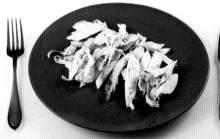

Weight: 160g

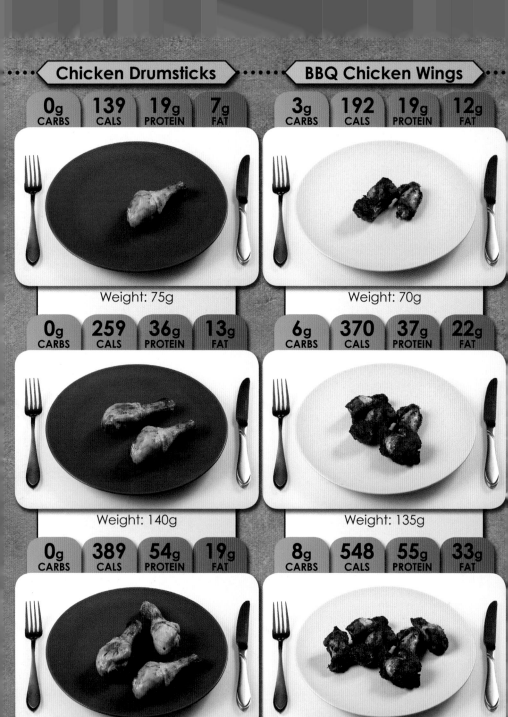

Chicken Drumsticks

| 0g CARBS | 139 CALS | 19g PROTEIN | 7g FAT |

Weight: 75g

| 0g CARBS | 259 CALS | 36g PROTEIN | 13g FAT |

Weight: 140g

| 0g CARBS | 389 CALS | 54g PROTEIN | 19g FAT |

Weight: 210g

BBQ Chicken Wings

| 3g CARBS | 192 CALS | 19g PROTEIN | 12g FAT |

Weight: 70g

| 6g CARBS | 370 CALS | 37g PROTEIN | 22g FAT |

Weight: 135g

| 8g CARBS | 548 CALS | 55g PROTEIN | 33g FAT |

Weight: 200g

Cod (baked)

0g CARBS	58 CALS	13g PROTEIN	1g FAT

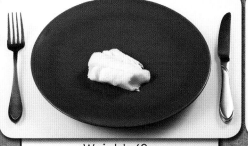

Weight: 60g

0g CARBS	120 CALS	27g PROTEIN	2g FAT

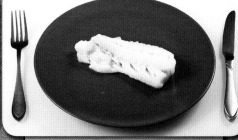

Weight: 125g

Tuna Steak (grilled)

0g CARBS	104 CALS	23g PROTEIN	1g FAT

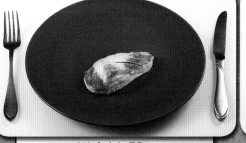

Weight: 75g

0g CARBS	181 CALS	39g PROTEIN	2g FAT

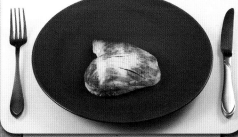

Weight: 130g

Trout Fillet (grilled)

0g CARBS	81 CALS	13g PROTEIN	3g FAT

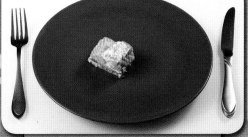

Weight: 60g

0g CARBS	142 CALS	23g PROTEIN	6g FAT

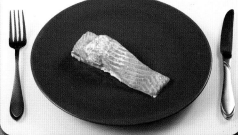

Weight: 105g

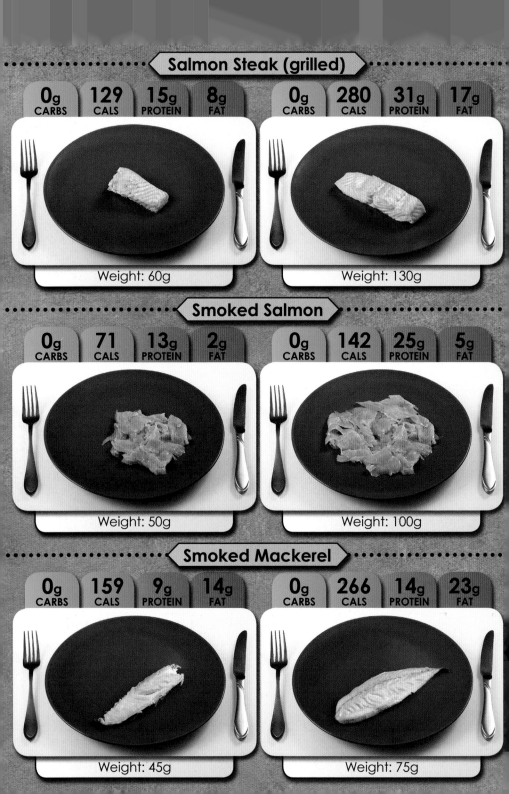

Salmon Steak (grilled)

0g CARBS	129 CALS	15g PROTEIN	8g FAT

Weight: 60g

0g CARBS	280 CALS	31g PROTEIN	17g FAT

Weight: 130g

Smoked Salmon

0g CARBS	71 CALS	13g PROTEIN	2g FAT

Weight: 50g

0g CARBS	142 CALS	25g PROTEIN	5g FAT

Weight: 100g

Smoked Mackerel

0g CARBS	159 CALS	9g PROTEIN	14g FAT

Weight: 45g

0g CARBS	266 CALS	14g PROTEIN	23g FAT

Weight: 75g

Prawns (boiled)

0g CARBS	50 CALS	11g PROTEIN	0g FAT

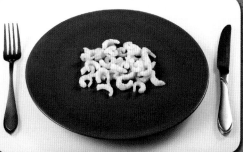

Weight: 50g

0g CARBS	99 CALS	23g PROTEIN	1g FAT

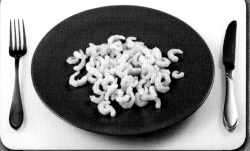

Weight: 100g

0g CARBS	149 CALS	34g PROTEIN	1g FAT

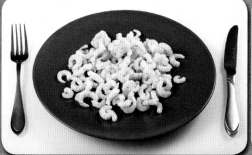

Weight: 150g

King Prawns (boiled)

0g CARBS	50 CALS	11g PROTEIN	0g FAT

Weight: 50g

0g CARBS	99 CALS	23g PROTEIN	1g FAT

Weight: 100g

0g CARBS	149 CALS	34g PROTEIN	1g FAT

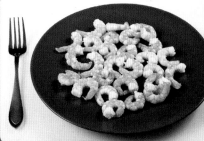

Weight: 150g

Tuna (tinned in brine)

0g CARBS	69 CALS	16g PROTEIN	0g FAT

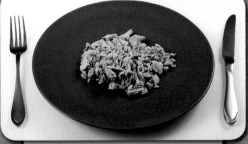

Weight: 70g (half tin)

0g CARBS	139 CALS	33g PROTEIN	1g FAT

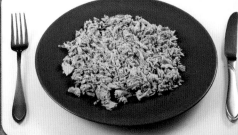

Weight: 140g (full tin)

Tuna (tinned in oil)

0g CARBS	132 CALS	19g PROTEIN	6g FAT

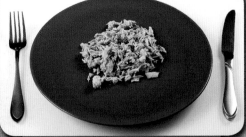

Weight: 70g (half tin)

0g CARBS	265 CALS	38g PROTEIN	13g FAT

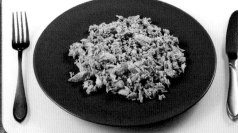

Weight: 140g (full tin)

Salmon (tinned in brine)

0g CARBS	142 CALS	18g PROTEIN	8g FAT

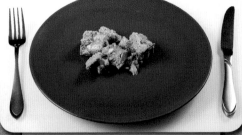

Weight: 85g (half tin)

0g CARBS	284 CALS	37g PROTEIN	15g FAT

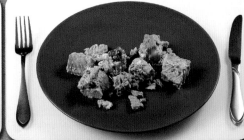

Weight: 170g (full tin)

Sardines (tinned in brine)

0g CARBS	86 CALS	11g PROTEIN	5g FAT

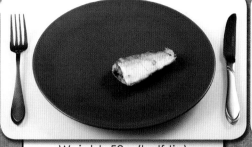

Weight: 50g (half tin)

0g CARBS	163 CALS	20g PROTEIN	9g FAT

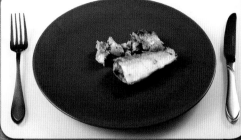

Weight: 95g (full tin)

Sardines (tinned in oil)

0g CARBS	110 CALS	12g PROTEIN	7g FAT

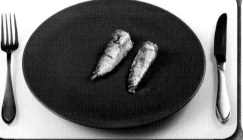

Weight: 50g (half tin)

0g CARBS	220 CALS	23g PROTEIN	14g FAT

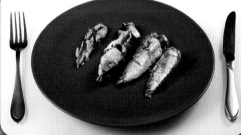

Weight: 100g (full tin)

Sardines (tinned in tomato sauce)

1g CARBS	81 CALS	9g PROTEIN	5g FAT

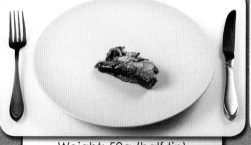

Weight: 50g (half tin)

1g CARBS	162 CALS	17g PROTEIN	10g FAT

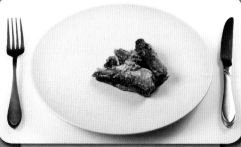

Weight: 100g (full tin)

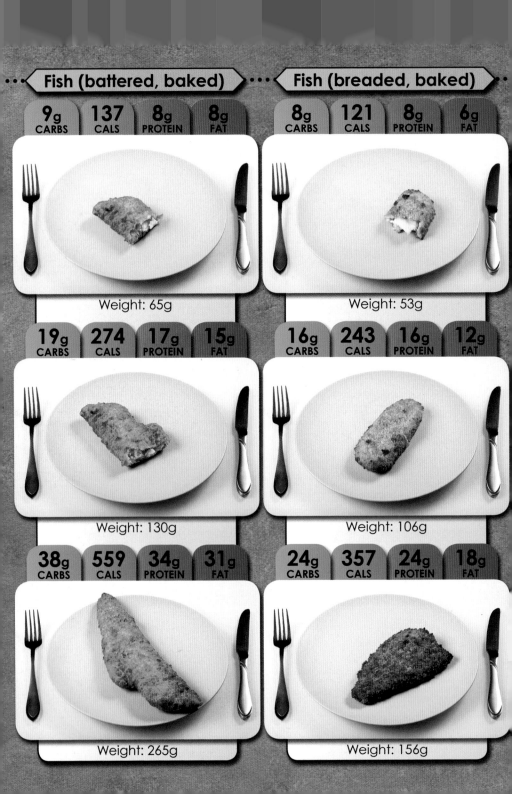

Fish (battered, baked)

| 9g CARBS | 137 CALS | 8g PROTEIN | 8g FAT |

Weight: 65g

| 19g CARBS | 274 CALS | 17g PROTEIN | 15g FAT |

Weight: 130g

| 38g CARBS | 559 CALS | 34g PROTEIN | 31g FAT |

Weight: 265g

Fish (breaded, baked)

| 8g CARBS | 121 CALS | 8g PROTEIN | 6g FAT |

Weight: 53g

| 16g CARBS | 243 CALS | 16g PROTEIN | 12g FAT |

Weight: 106g

| 24g CARBS | 357 CALS | 24g PROTEIN | 18g FAT |

Weight: 156g

Fish Cake (baked)

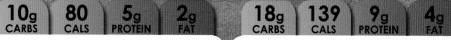

| 10g CARBS | 80 CALS | 5g PROTEIN | 2g FAT |

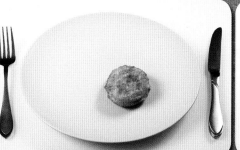

	CARBS	CALS	PROT	FAT
2x	20g	160	10g	4g
3x	30g	240	15g	6g
4x	40g	320	20g	8g

Weight: 52g

| 18g CARBS | 139 CALS | 9g PROTEIN | 4g FAT |

	CARBS	CALS	PROT	FAT
2x	36g	278	18g	8g
3x	54g	417	27g	12g
4x	72g	556	36g	16g

Weight: 90g

Fish Finger (grilled)

| 3g CARBS | 40 CALS | 3g PROTEIN | 2g FAT |

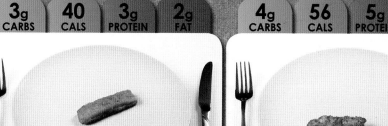

	CARBS	CALS	PROT	FAT
2x	6g	80	6g	4g
3x	9g	120	9g	6g
4x	12g	160	12g	8g

Weight: 20g

Fish Goujon (baked)

| 4g CARBS | 56 CALS | 5g PROTEIN | 4g FAT |

	CARBS	CALS	PROT	FAT
2x	8g	112	10g	8g
3x	12g	168	15g	12g
4x	16g	224	20g	16g

Weight: 30g

Scampi (fried)

14g CARBS	166 CALS	7g PROTEIN	10g FAT

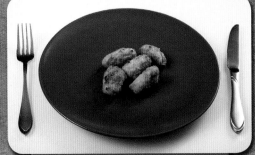

Weight: 70g

29g CARBS	332 CALS	13g PROTEIN	19g FAT

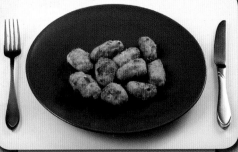

Weight: 140g

43g CARBS	493 CALS	20g PROTEIN	28g FAT

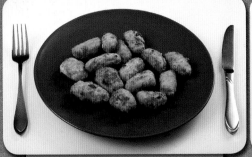

Weight: 208g

Haggis

20g CARBS	326 CALS	11g PROTEIN	23g FAT

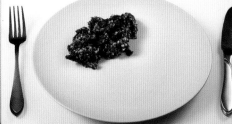

Weight: 105g

40g CARBS	651 CALS	22g PROTEIN	46g FAT

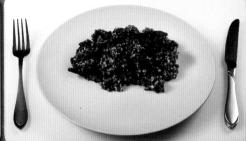

Weight: 210g

60g CARBS	977 CALS	34g PROTEIN	68g FAT

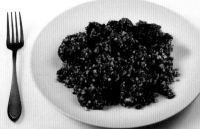

Weight: 315g

Chicken Kiev (baked)

15g CARBS	348 CALS	24g PROTEIN	22g FAT

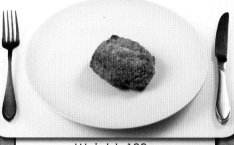

Weight: 130g

30g CARBS	697 CALS	48g PROTEIN	44g FAT

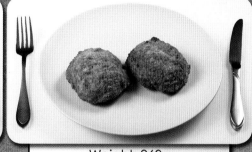

Weight: 260g

Pork Pie

28g CARBS	432 CALS	13g PROTEIN	31g FAT

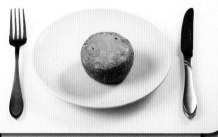

Weight: 119g

76g CARBS	1162 CALS	35g PROTEIN	82g FAT

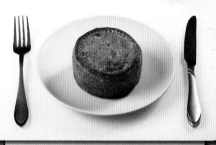

Weight: 320g

Scotch Egg

8g CARBS	145 CALS	7g PROTEIN	10g FAT

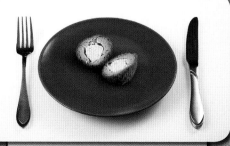

Weight: 60g

16g CARBS	289 CALS	14g PROTEIN	19g FAT

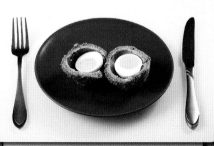

Weight: 120g

8g CARBS	83 CALS	2g PROTEIN	5g FAT

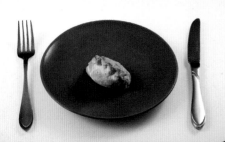

Weight: 31g

41g CARBS	433 CALS	11g PROTEIN	26g FAT

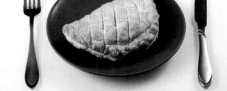

Weight: 162g

49g CARBS	518 CALS	13g PROTEIN	32g FAT

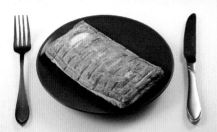

Weight: 194g

109g CARBS	1159 CALS	29g PROTEIN	71g FAT

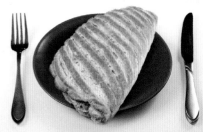

Weight: 434g

16g CARBS	241 CALS	6g PROTEIN	17g FAT

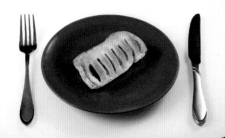

Weight: 63g

31g CARBS	475 CALS	12g PROTEIN	34g FAT

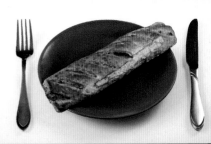

Weight: 124g

Sausages & Beans (tinned)

10g CARBS	76 CALS	4g PROTEIN	2g FAT

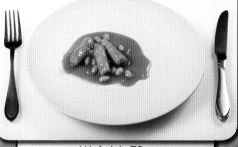

Weight: 70g

20g CARBS	153 CALS	8g PROTEIN	5g FAT

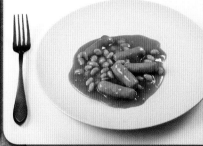

Weight: 140g

30g CARBS	229 CALS	12g PROTEIN	7g FAT

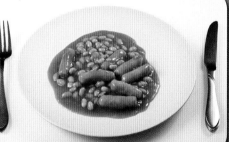
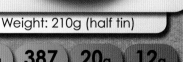

Weight: 210g (half tin)

40g CARBS	311 CALS	16g PROTEIN	9g FAT

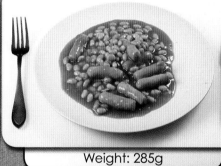

Weight: 285g

50g CARBS	387 CALS	20g PROTEIN	12g FAT

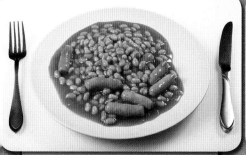

Weight: 355g

60g CARBS	463 CALS	24g PROTEIN	14g FAT

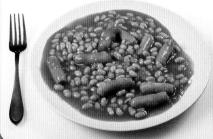

Weight: 425g (full tin)

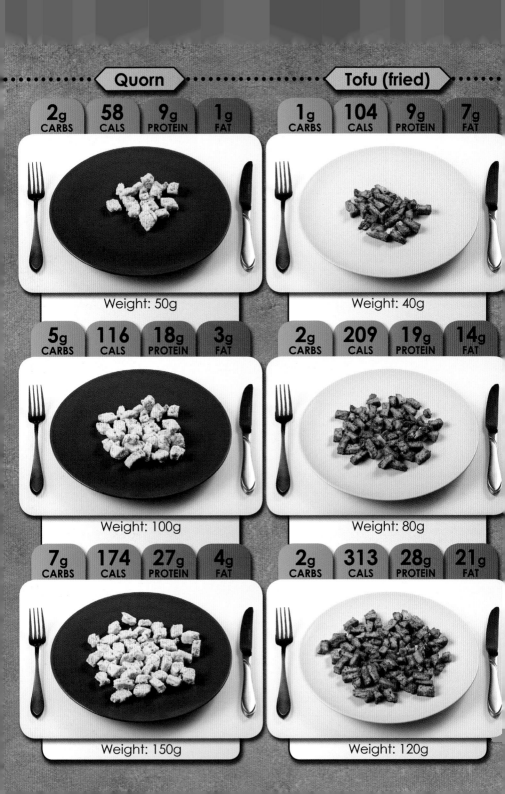

Quorn

| 2g CARBS | 58 CALS | 9g PROTEIN | 1g FAT |

Weight: 50g

| 5g CARBS | 116 CALS | 18g PROTEIN | 3g FAT |

Weight: 100g

| 7g CARBS | 174 CALS | 27g PROTEIN | 4g FAT |

Weight: 150g

Tofu (fried)

| 1g CARBS | 104 CALS | 9g PROTEIN | 7g FAT |

Weight: 40g

| 2g CARBS | 209 CALS | 19g PROTEIN | 14g FAT |

Weight: 80g

| 2g CARBS | 313 CALS | 28g PROTEIN | 21g FAT |

Weight: 120g

Cassava Chips (deep fried)

23g CARBS	122 CALS	0g PROTEIN	3g FAT

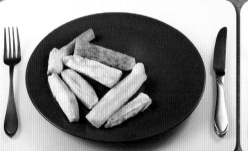

Weight: 45g

47g CARBS	246 CALS	1g PROTEIN	5g FAT

Weight: 91g

71g CARBS	367 CALS	1g PROTEIN	8g FAT

Weight: 136g

95g CARBS	491 CALS	2g PROTEIN	11g FAT

Weight: 182g

119g CARBS	616 CALS	2g PROTEIN	14g FAT

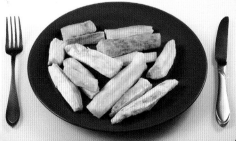

Weight: 228g

141g CARBS	734 CALS	3g PROTEIN	16g FAT

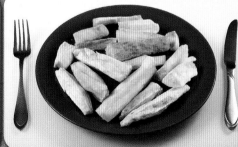

Weight: 272g

Chips (deep fried)

12g CARBS	90 CALS	1g PROTEIN	4g FAT

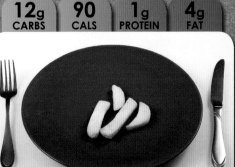

Weight: 33g

36g CARBS	270 CALS	4g PROTEIN	13g FAT

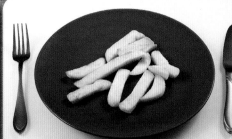

Weight: 99g

59g CARBS	450 CALS	7g PROTEIN	22g FAT

Weight: 165g

83g CARBS	628 CALS	9g PROTEIN	31g FAT

Weight: 230g

106g CARBS	805 CALS	12g PROTEIN	40g FAT

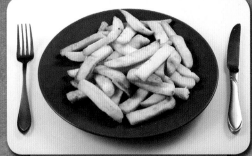

Weight: 295g

130g CARBS	983 CALS	15g PROTEIN	49g FAT

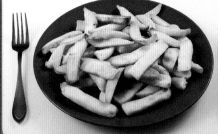

Weight: 360g

Chips (oven)

10g CARBS	53 CALS	1g PROTEIN	1g FAT

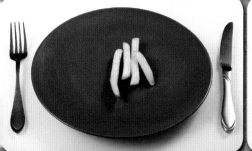

Weight: 33g

30g CARBS	162 CALS	3g PROTEIN	4g FAT

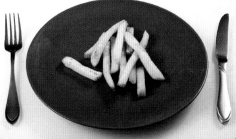

Weight: 100g

50g CARBS	272 CALS	5g PROTEIN	7g FAT

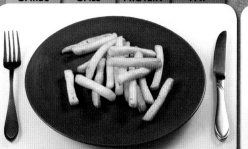

Weight: 168g

70g CARBS	381 CALS	8g PROTEIN	10g FAT

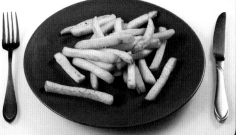

Weight: 235g

90g CARBS	491 CALS	10g PROTEIN	13g FAT

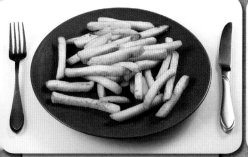

Weight: 303g

110g CARBS	599 CALS	12g PROTEIN	16g FAT

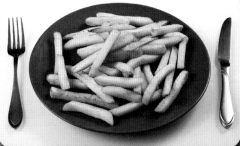

Weight: 370g

Dauphinoise Potatoes

10g CARBS	178 CALS	2g PROTEIN	15g FAT

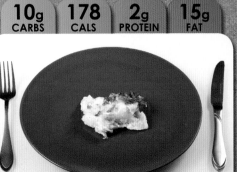

Weight: 72g

20g CARBS	363 CALS	4g PROTEIN	31g FAT

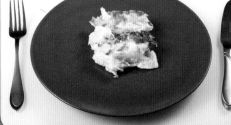

Weight: 147g

30g CARBS	548 CALS	5g PROTEIN	46g FAT

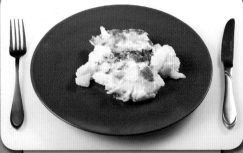

Weight: 222g

40g CARBS	734 CALS	7g PROTEIN	62g FAT

Weight: 297g

50g CARBS	921 CALS	9g PROTEIN	78g FAT

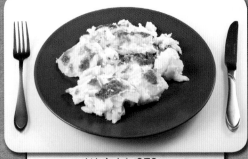

Weight: 373g

60g CARBS	1107 CALS	11g PROTEIN	93g FAT

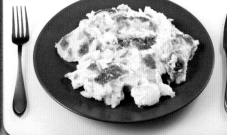

Weight: 448g

Gnocchi

27g CARBS	122 CALS	3g PROTEIN	0g FAT

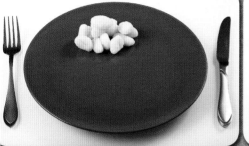

Weight: 80g

55g CARBS	245 CALS	6g PROTEIN	0g FAT

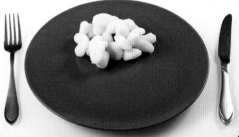

Weight: 160g

82g CARBS	367 CALS	9g PROTEIN	1g FAT

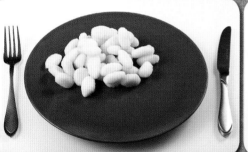

Weight: 240g

110g CARBS	493 CALS	12g PROTEIN	1g FAT

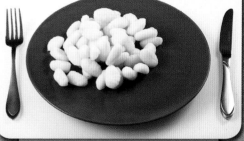

Weight: 322g

137g CARBS	615 CALS	14g PROTEIN	1g FAT

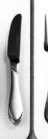

Weight: 402g

164g CARBS	737 CALS	17g PROTEIN	1g FAT

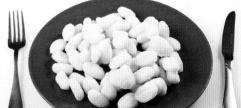

Weight: 482g

Jacket Potato (baked with skin)

| 20g CARBS | 90 CALS | 3g PROTEIN | 0g FAT |

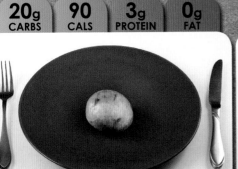

Weight: 95g

| 35g CARBS | 152 CALS | 4g PROTEIN | 0g FAT |

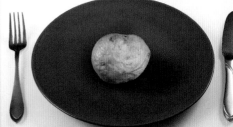
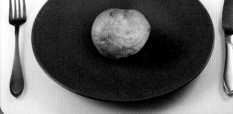
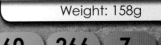

Weight: 158g

| 45g CARBS | 200 CALS | 6g PROTEIN | 1g FAT |

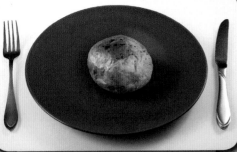
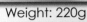

Weight: 220g

| 60g CARBS | 266 CALS | 7g PROTEIN | 1g FAT |

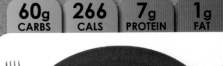
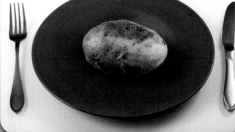

Weight: 284g

| 75g CARBS | 333 CALS | 9g PROTEIN | 1g FAT |

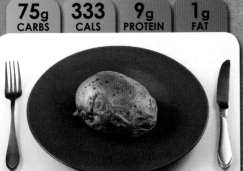

Weight: 348g

| 90g CARBS | 386 CALS | 11g PROTEIN | 1g FAT |

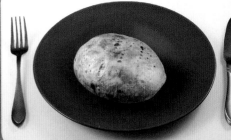

Weight: 410g

Mashed Potato (with butter)

19g CARBS	125 CALS	2g PROTEIN	5g FAT

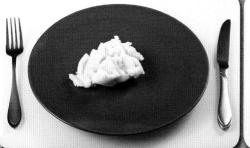

Weight: 120g

36g CARBS	244 CALS	4g PROTEIN	10g FAT

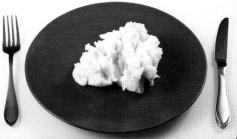

Weight: 235g

55g CARBS	369 CALS	6g PROTEIN	15g FAT

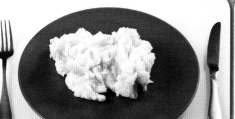

Weight: 355g

73g CARBS	489 CALS	8g PROTEIN	20g FAT

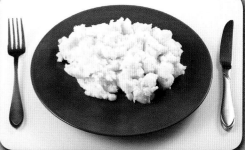

Weight: 470g

91g CARBS	614 CALS	11g PROTEIN	25g FAT

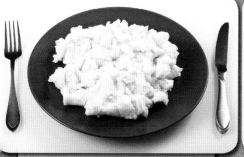

Weight: 590g

109g CARBS	733 CALS	13g PROTEIN	30g FAT

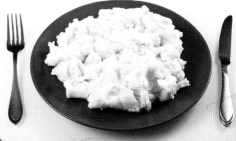

Weight: 705g

New Potatoes (boiled)

10g CARBS	43 CALS	1g PROTEIN	0g FAT

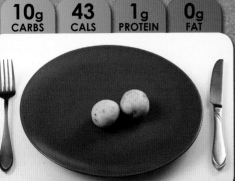

Weight: 65g

20g CARBS	86 CALS	2g PROTEIN	0g FAT

Weight: 130g

30g CARBS	129 CALS	3g PROTEIN	1g FAT

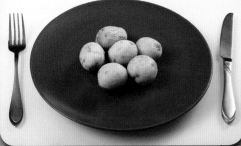

Weight: 195g

40g CARBS	172 CALS	4g PROTEIN	1g FAT

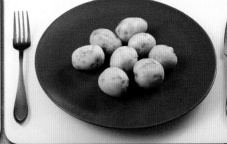

Weight: 260g

60g CARBS	257 CALS	5g PROTEIN	1g FAT

Weight: 390g

80g CARBS	343 CALS	7g PROTEIN	2g FAT

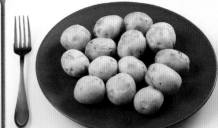

Weight: 520g

Potato Faces (baked)

10g CARBS	72 CALS	1g PROTEIN	3g FAT

Weight: 34g

21g CARBS	145 CALS	2g PROTEIN	6g FAT

Weight: 68g

31g CARBS	217 CALS	3g PROTEIN	9g FAT

Weight: 102g

42g CARBS	290 CALS	4g PROTEIN	12g FAT

Weight: 136g

52g CARBS	362 CALS	5g PROTEIN	15g FAT

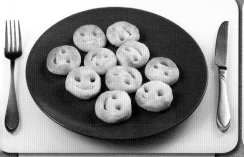

Weight: 170g

63g CARBS	435 CALS	6g PROTEIN	18g FAT

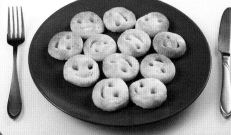

Weight: 204g

Roast Potatoes

10g CARBS	57 CALS	1g PROTEIN	2g FAT

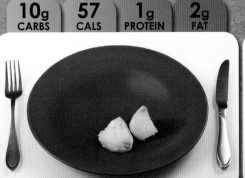

Weight: 38g

25g CARBS	142 CALS	3g PROTEIN	4g FAT

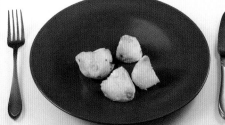

Weight: 95g

40g CARBS	231 CALS	4g PROTEIN	7g FAT

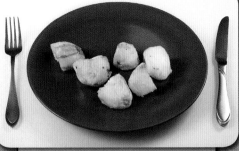

Weight: 155g

55g CARBS	316 CALS	6g PROTEIN	10g FAT

Weight: 212g

70g CARBS	402 CALS	8g PROTEIN	12g FAT

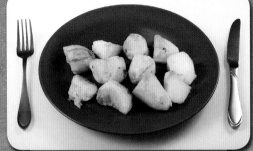

Weight: 270g

85g CARBS	492 CALS	10g PROTEIN	15g FAT

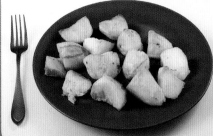

Weight: 330g

Sauté Potatoes (baked)

| **10**g CARBS | **56** CALS | **1**g PROTEIN | **1**g FAT |

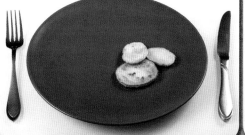

Weight: 28g

| **20**g CARBS | **109** CALS | **2**g PROTEIN | **2**g FAT |

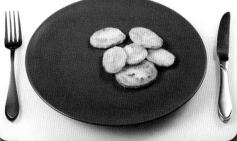

Weight: 55g

| **30**g CARBS | **159** CALS | **4**g PROTEIN | **3**g FAT |

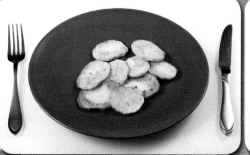

Weight: 80g

| **40**g CARBS | **215** CALS | **5**g PROTEIN | **4**g FAT |

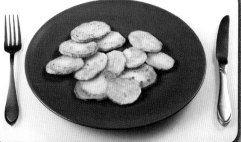

Weight: 108g

| **50**g CARBS | **269** CALS | **6**g PROTEIN | **5**g FAT |

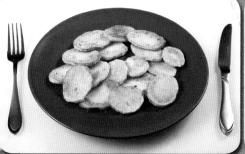

Weight: 135g

| **60**g CARBS | **322** CALS | **7**g PROTEIN | **6**g FAT |

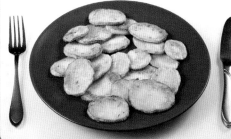

Weight: 162g

Sweet Potatoes (baked)

15g CARBS	63 CALS	1g PROTEIN	0g FAT

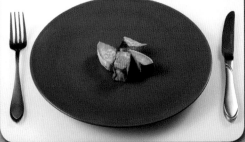

Weight: 55g

30g CARBS	124 CALS	2g PROTEIN	0g FAT

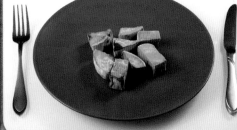

Weight: 108g

45g CARBS	184 CALS	3g PROTEIN	1g FAT

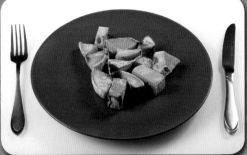

Weight: 160g

60g CARBS	247 CALS	3g PROTEIN	1g FAT

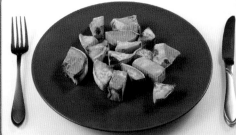

Weight: 215g

75g CARBS	311 CALS	4g PROTEIN	1g FAT

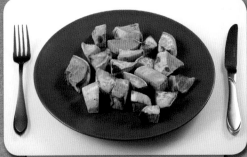

Weight: 270g

90g CARBS	370 CALS	5g PROTEIN	1g FAT

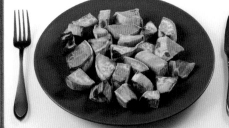

Weight: 322g

Wedges (baked)

13g CARBS	78 CALS	1g PROTEIN	3g FAT

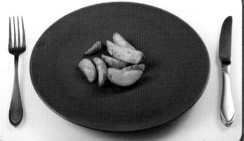

Weight: 55g

25g CARBS	156 CALS	2g PROTEIN	5g FAT

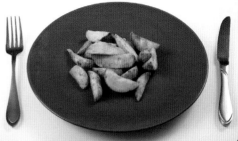

Weight: 110g

38g CARBS	234 CALS	3g PROTEIN	8g FAT

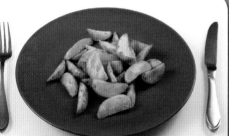

Weight: 165g

51g CARBS	312 CALS	4g PROTEIN	10g FAT

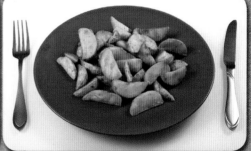

Weight: 220g

62g CARBS	383 CALS	5g PROTEIN	13g FAT

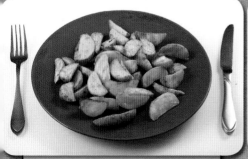

Weight: 270g

75g CARBS	462 CALS	7g PROTEIN	15g FAT

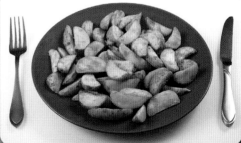

Weight: 325g

Hash Brown (baked)

10g CARBS	83 CALS	1g PROTEIN	4g FAT

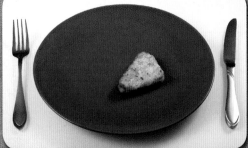

	CARBS	CALS	PROT	FAT
2x	20g	166	2g	8g
3x	30g	249	3g	12g
4x	40g	332	4g	16g
Weight: 44g				

Potato Croquette (fried)

5g CARBS	47 CALS	1g PROTEIN	3g FAT

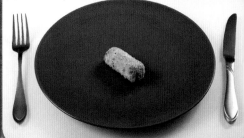

	CARBS	CALS	PROT	FAT
2x	10g	94	2g	6g
3x	15g	141	3g	9g
4x	20g	188	4g	12g
Weight: 22g				

Potato Rosti (baked)

20g CARBS	155 CALS	2g PROTEIN	7g FAT

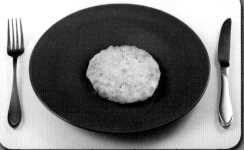

	CARBS	CALS	PROT	FAT
2x	40g	310	4g	14g
3x	60g	465	6g	21g
4x	80g	620	8g	28g
Weight: 80g				

Potato Waffle (baked)

15g CARBS	119 CALS	2g PROTEIN	6g FAT

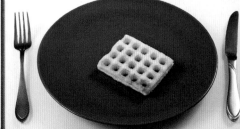

	CARBS	CALS	PROT	FAT
2x	30g	238	4g	12g
3x	45g	357	6g	18g
4x	60g	476	8g	24g
Weight: 49g				

Bulgar Wheat

20g CARBS	**94** CALS	**3**g PROTEIN	**0**g FAT

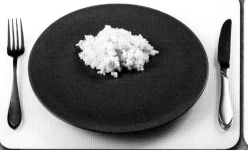

Weight: 100g

40g CARBS	**188** CALS	**5**g PROTEIN	**1**g FAT

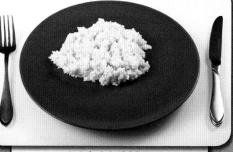

Weight: 200g

60g CARBS	**277** CALS	**7**g PROTEIN	**1**g FAT

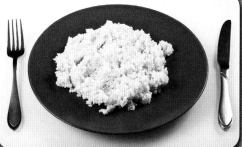

Weight: 295g

Quinoa

20g CARBS	**109** CALS	**5**g PROTEIN	**2**g FAT

Weight: 85g

40g CARBS	**220** CALS	**10**g PROTEIN	**4**g FAT

Weight: 172g

60g CARBS	**333** CALS	**15**g PROTEIN	**5**g FAT

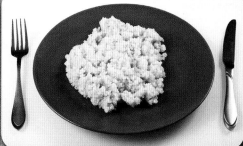

Weight: 260g

COUSCOUS

10g CARBS	**50** CALS	**1g** PROTEIN	**0g** FAT

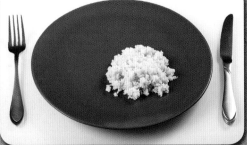

Weight: 45g

25g CARBS	**121** CALS	**3g** PROTEIN	**1g** FAT

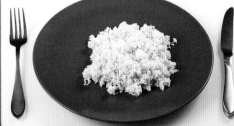

Weight: 110g

40g CARBS	**193** CALS	**5g** PROTEIN	**1g** FAT

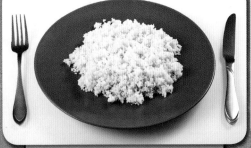

Weight: 175g

55g CARBS	**264** CALS	**6g** PROTEIN	**1g** FAT

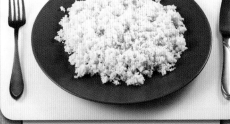

Weight: 240g

70g CARBS	**336** CALS	**8g** PROTEIN	**2g** FAT

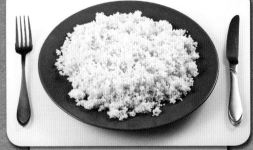

Weight: 305g

85g CARBS	**407** CALS	**10g** PROTEIN	**2g** FAT

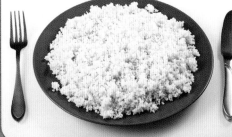

Weight: 370g

Noodles (egg)

20g CARBS	101 CALS	3g PROTEIN	2g FAT

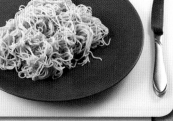

Weight: 58g

40g CARBS	200 CALS	6g PROTEIN	4g FAT

Weight: 115g

60g CARBS	296 CALS	10g PROTEIN	6g FAT

Weight: 170g

80g CARBS	397 CALS	13g PROTEIN	9g FAT

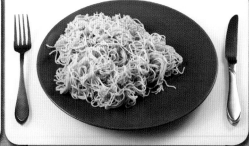

Weight: 228g

100g CARBS	496 CALS	16g PROTEIN	11g FAT

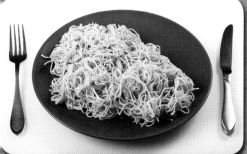

Weight: 285g

120g CARBS	595 CALS	19g PROTEIN	13g FAT

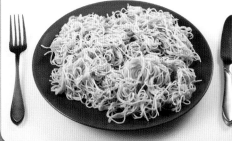

Weight: 342g

Noodles (rice)

20g CARBS	**86** CALS	**1g** PROTEIN	**0g** FAT

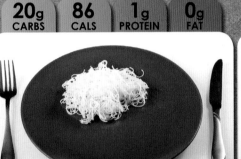

Weight: 70g

40g CARBS	**175** CALS	**2g** PROTEIN	**0g** FAT

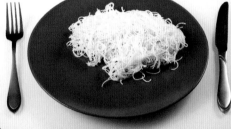

Weight: 142g

60g CARBS	**264** CALS	**4g** PROTEIN	**0g** FAT

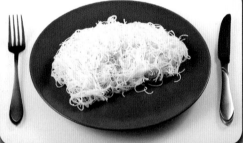

Weight: 215g

80g CARBS	**351** CALS	**5g** PROTEIN	**0g** FAT

Weight: 285g

100g CARBS	**440** CALS	**6g** PROTEIN	**0g** FAT

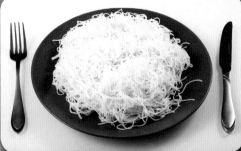

Weight: 358g

120g CARBS	**529** CALS	**7g** PROTEIN	**0g** FAT

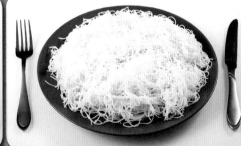

Weight: 430g

Pasta (bows)

10g CARBS	50 CALS	2g PROTEIN	0g FAT

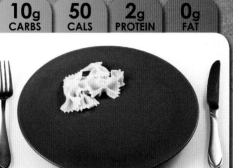

Weight: 30g

30g CARBS	148 CALS	5g PROTEIN	1g FAT

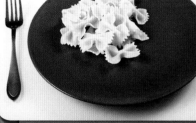

Weight: 88g

50g CARBS	249 CALS	8g PROTEIN	1g FAT

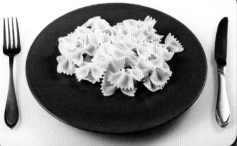

Weight: 148g

70g CARBS	344 CALS	11g PROTEIN	2g FAT

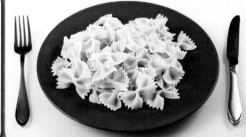

Weight: 205g

90g CARBS	445 CALS	14g PROTEIN	3g FAT

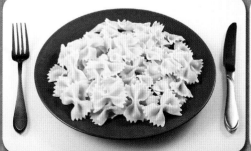

Weight: 265g

110g CARBS	543 CALS	17g PROTEIN	3g FAT

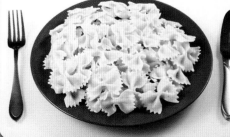

Weight: 323g

Pasta (macaroni)

10g CARBS	49 CALS	2g PROTEIN	0g FAT		30g CARBS	152 CALS	5g PROTEIN	1g FAT

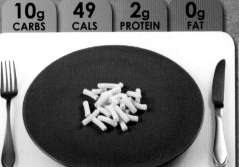

Weight: 32g

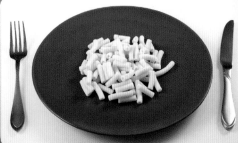

Weight: 100g

50g CARBS	252 CALS	9g PROTEIN	2g FAT		70g CARBS	354 CALS	12g PROTEIN	2g FAT

Weight: 166g

Weight: 233g

90g CARBS	456 CALS	16g PROTEIN	3g FAT		110g CARBS	556 CALS	19g PROTEIN	4g FAT

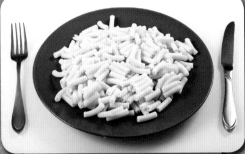

Weight: 300g

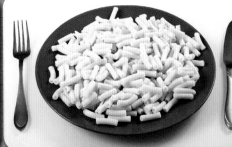

Weight: 366g

Pasta (penne)

| 10g CARBS | 50 CALS | 2g PROTEIN | 0g FAT |

Weight: 30g

| 30g CARBS | 150 CALS | 5g PROTEIN | 1g FAT |

Weight: 90g

| 50g CARBS | 247 CALS | 8g PROTEIN | 1g FAT |

Weight: 148g

| 70g CARBS | 347 CALS | 11g PROTEIN | 2g FAT |

Weight: 208g

| 90g CARBS | 443 CALS | 14g PROTEIN | 3g FAT |

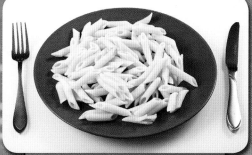

Weight: 265g

| 110g CARBS | 543 CALS | 17g PROTEIN | 3g FAT |

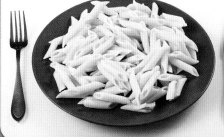

Weight: 325g

Pasta (shells)

10g CARBS	50 CALS	2g PROTEIN	0g FAT

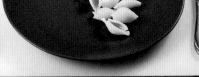

Weight: 30g

30g CARBS	147 CALS	5g PROTEIN	1g FAT

Weight: 88g

50g CARBS	247 CALS	8g PROTEIN	1g FAT

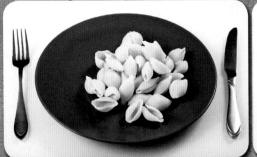

Weight: 148g

70g CARBS	342 CALS	11g PROTEIN	2g FAT

Weight: 205g

90g CARBS	443 CALS	14g PROTEIN	3g FAT

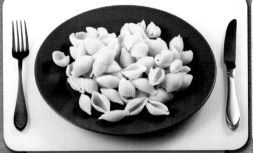

Weight: 265g

110g CARBS	539 CALS	17g PROTEIN	3g FAT

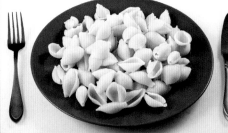

Weight: 323g

Pasta (tagliatelle)

10g CARBS	53 CALS	2g PROTEIN	0g FAT

Weight: 30g

30g CARBS	158 CALS	5g PROTEIN	1g FAT

Weight: 90g

50g CARBS	263 CALS	8g PROTEIN	2g FAT

Weight: 150g

70g CARBS	368 CALS	11g PROTEIN	2g FAT

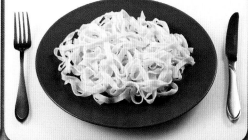

Weight: 210g

90g CARBS	473 CALS	14g PROTEIN	3g FAT

Weight: 270g

110g CARBS	578 CALS	17g PROTEIN	3g FAT

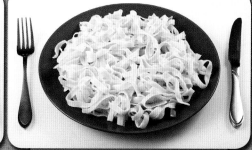

Weight: 330g

Pasta (twirls)

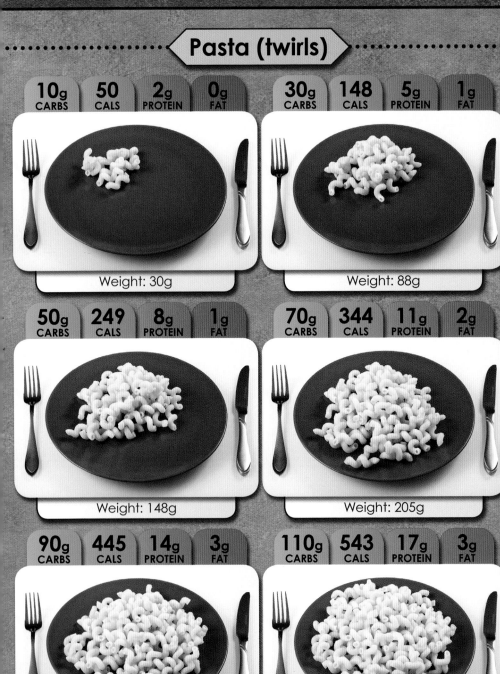

10g CARBS	50 CALS	2g PROTEIN	0g FAT

Weight: 30g

30g CARBS	148 CALS	5g PROTEIN	1g FAT

Weight: 88g

50g CARBS	249 CALS	8g PROTEIN	1g FAT

Weight: 148g

70g CARBS	344 CALS	11g PROTEIN	2g FAT

Weight: 205g

90g CARBS	445 CALS	14g PROTEIN	3g FAT

Weight: 265g

110g CARBS	543 CALS	17g PROTEIN	3g FAT

Weight: 323g

Pasta (twists)

10g CARBS	51 CALS	2g PROTEIN	0g FAT

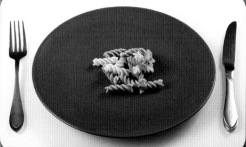

Weight: 30g

30g CARBS	149 CALS	5g PROTEIN	1g FAT

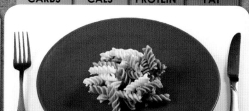

Weight: 88g

50g CARBS	245 CALS	8g PROTEIN	1g FAT

Weight: 145g

70g CARBS	343 CALS	11g PROTEIN	2g FAT

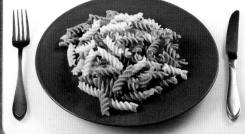

Weight: 203g

90g CARBS	439 CALS	14g PROTEIN	3g FAT

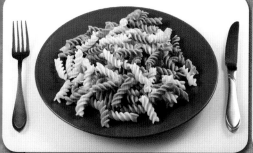

Weight: 260g

110g CARBS	537 CALS	17g PROTEIN	3g FAT

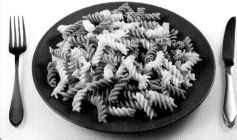

Weight: 318g

Pasta (vermicelli)

10g CARBS	52 CALS	2g PROTEIN	1g FAT

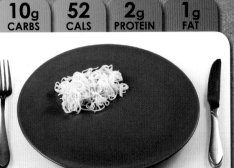

Weight: 40g

30g CARBS	161 CALS	6g PROTEIN	2g FAT

Weight: 125g

50g CARBS	271 CALS	11g PROTEIN	3g FAT

Weight: 210g

70g CARBS	374 CALS	15g PROTEIN	4g FAT

Weight: 290g

90g CARBS	484 CALS	19g PROTEIN	5g FAT

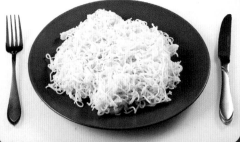

Weight: 375g

110g CARBS	593 CALS	23g PROTEIN	6g FAT

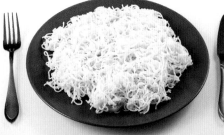

Weight: 460g

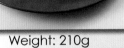
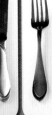

Rice (white)

| 10g CARBS | 44 CALS | 1g PROTEIN | 0g FAT |

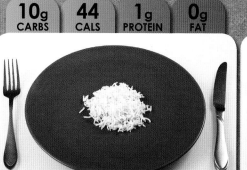

Weight: 32g

| 30g CARBS | 132 CALS | 2g PROTEIN | 1g FAT |

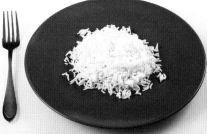

Weight: 96g

| 50g CARBS | 225 CALS | 4g PROTEIN | 2g FAT |

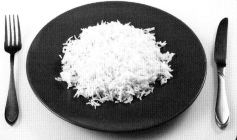

Weight: 163g

| 70g CARBS | 311 CALS | 6g PROTEIN | 3g FAT |

Weight: 225g

| 90g CARBS | 400 CALS | 8g PROTEIN | 4g FAT |

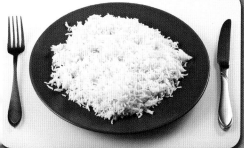

Weight: 290g

| 110g CARBS | 490 CALS | 9g PROTEIN | 5g FAT |

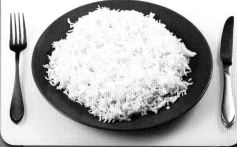

Weight: 355g

Rice (brown)

10g CARBS	42 CALS	1g PROTEIN	0g FAT

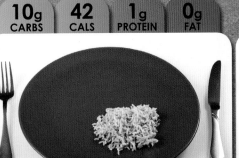

Weight: 30g

30g CARBS	134 CALS	2g PROTEIN	1g FAT

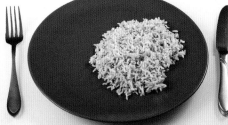

Weight: 95g

50g CARBS	219 CALS	4g PROTEIN	2g FAT

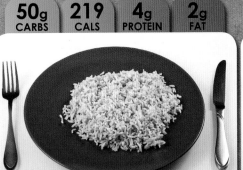

Weight: 155g

70g CARBS	307 CALS	6g PROTEIN	2g FAT

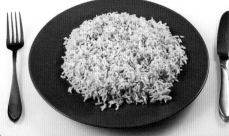

Weight: 218g

90g CARBS	395 CALS	7g PROTEIN	3g FAT

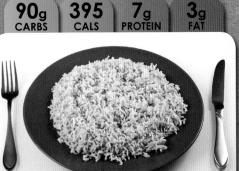

Weight: 280g

110g CARBS	484 CALS	9g PROTEIN	4g FAT

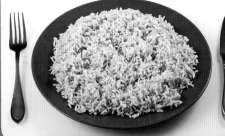

Weight: 343g

Rice (sticky white)

21g CARBS	110 CALS	2g PROTEIN	2g FAT

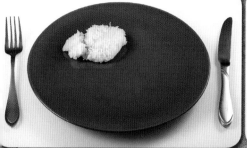

Weight: 80g

Polenta

10g CARBS	47 CALS	1g PROTEIN	0g FAT

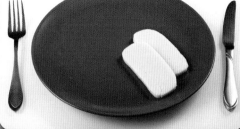

Weight: 65g

41g CARBS	212 CALS	4g PROTEIN	3g FAT

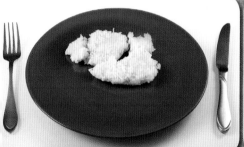

Weight: 155g

20g CARBS	94 CALS	2g PROTEIN	0g FAT

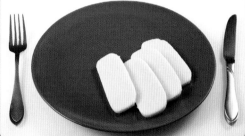

Weight: 130g

63g CARBS	322 CALS	6g PROTEIN	5g FAT

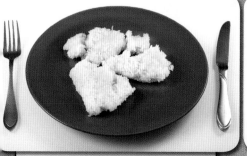

Weight: 235g

30g CARBS	137 CALS	3g PROTEIN	1g FAT

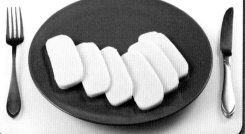

Weight: 190g

Ravioli (fresh, meat-filled)

10g CARBS	71 CALS	3g PROTEIN	2g FAT

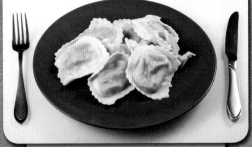

Weight: 40g

30g CARBS	204 CALS	9g PROTEIN	5g FAT

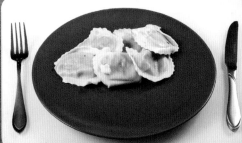

Weight: 115g

50g CARBS	340 CALS	16g PROTEIN	8g FAT

Weight: 192g

70g CARBS	478 CALS	22g PROTEIN	12g FAT

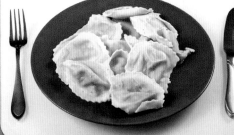

Weight: 270g

90g CARBS	611 CALS	28g PROTEIN	15g FAT

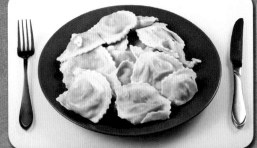

Weight: 345g

110g CARBS	747 CALS	35g PROTEIN	19g FAT

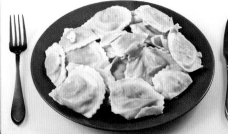

Weight: 422g

Spaghetti (white)

10g CARBS	52 CALS	2g PROTEIN	0g FAT

Weight: 33g

30g CARBS	149 CALS	5g PROTEIN	1g FAT

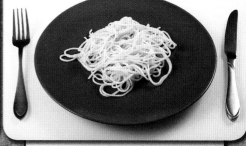

Weight: 95g

50g CARBS	248 CALS	8g PROTEIN	2g FAT

Weight: 158g

70g CARBS	345 CALS	12g PROTEIN	2g FAT

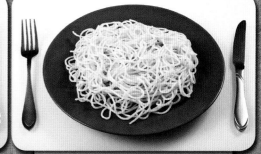

Weight: 220g

90g CARBS	447 CALS	15g PROTEIN	3g FAT

Weight: 285g

110g CARBS	546 CALS	18g PROTEIN	3g FAT

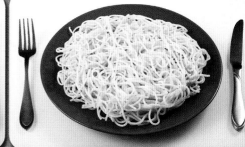

Weight: 348g

Spaghetti (wholemeal)

10g CARBS	48 CALS	2g PROTEIN	0g FAT

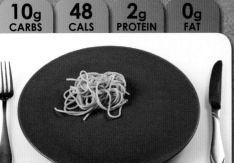

Weight: 33g

30g CARBS	151 CALS	6g PROTEIN	1g FAT

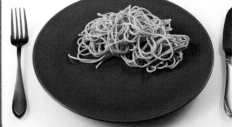

Weight: 105g

50g CARBS	248 CALS	9g PROTEIN	2g FAT

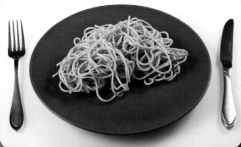

Weight: 172g

70g CARBS	346 CALS	13g PROTEIN	2g FAT

Weight: 240g

90g CARBS	446 CALS	16g PROTEIN	3g FAT

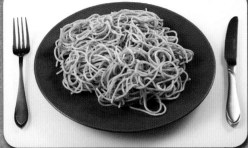

Weight: 310g

110g CARBS	547 CALS	20g PROTEIN	4g FAT

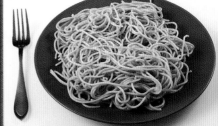

Weight: 380g

Tortellini (fresh, cheese-filled)

13g CARBS	91 CALS	4g PROTEIN	3g FAT

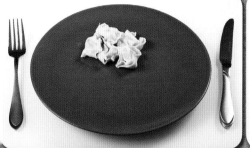

Weight: 42g

45g CARBS	308 CALS	13g PROTEIN	9g FAT

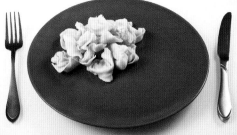

Weight: 142g

76g CARBS	525 CALS	23g PROTEIN	15g FAT

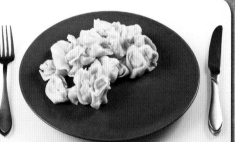

Weight: 242g

107g CARBS	742 CALS	32g PROTEIN	21g FAT

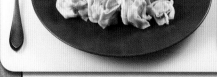

Weight: 342g

139g CARBS	959 CALS	41g PROTEIN	27g FAT

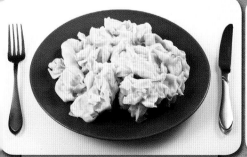

Weight: 442g

170g CARBS	1176 CALS	50g PROTEIN	33g FAT

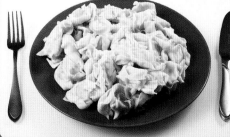

Weight: 542g

Pasta Shapes (tinned)

9g CARBS	**42** CALS	**1g** PROTEIN	**0g** FAT

Weight: 70g

17g CARBS	**84** CALS	**3g** PROTEIN	**1g** FAT

Weight: 140g

26g CARBS	**126** CALS	**4g** PROTEIN	**1g** FAT

Weight: 210g (half tin)

35g CARBS	**171** CALS	**5g** PROTEIN	**1g** FAT

Weight: 285g

44g CARBS	**213** CALS	**6g** PROTEIN	**1g** FAT

Weight: 355g

52g CARBS	**255** CALS	**8g** PROTEIN	**2g** FAT

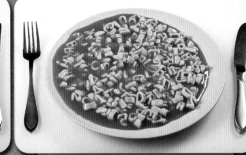

Weight: 425g (full tin)

Ravioli in Tomato Sauce (tinned)

7g CARBS	49 CALS	2g PROTEIN	2g FAT

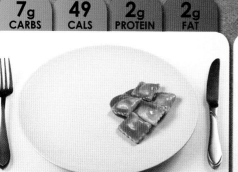

Weight: 70g

14g CARBS	98 CALS	4g PROTEIN	3g FAT

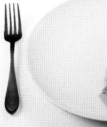

Weight: 140g

22g CARBS	147 CALS	6g PROTEIN	5g FAT

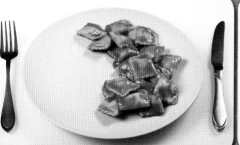

Weight: 210g (half tin)

29g CARBS	200 CALS	9g PROTEIN	6g FAT

Weight: 285g

37g CARBS	249 CALS	11g PROTEIN	8g FAT

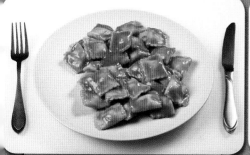

Weight: 355g

44g CARBS	298 CALS	13g PROTEIN	9g FAT

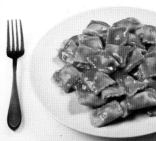

Weight: 425g (full tin)

Spaghetti in Tomato Sauce (tinned)

10g CARBS	45 CALS	1g PROTEIN	0g FAT

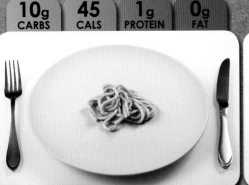

Weight: 70g

20g CARBS	90 CALS	3g PROTEIN	1g FAT

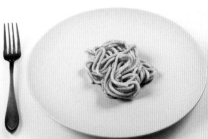

Weight: 140g

30g CARBS	134 CALS	4g PROTEIN	1g FAT

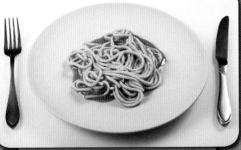

Weight: 210g (half tin)

40g CARBS	182 CALS	5g PROTEIN	1g FAT

Weight: 285g

50g CARBS	227 CALS	7g PROTEIN	1g FAT

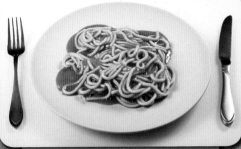

Weight: 355g

60g CARBS	272 CALS	8g PROTEIN	2g FAT

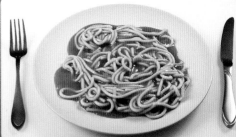

Weight: 425g (full tin)

Spaghetti Hoops in Tomato Sauce (tinned)

9g CARBS	41 CALS	1g PROTEIN	0g FAT

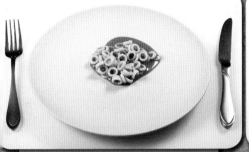

Weight: 70g

17g CARBS	81 CALS	2g PROTEIN	0g FAT

Weight: 140g

26g CARBS	122 CALS	4g PROTEIN	0g FAT

Weight: 210g (half tin)

34g CARBS	162 CALS	5g PROTEIN	1g FAT

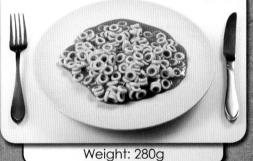

Weight: 280g

43g CARBS	203 CALS	6g PROTEIN	1g FAT

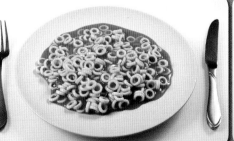

Weight: 350g

52g CARBS	244 CALS	7g PROTEIN	1g FAT

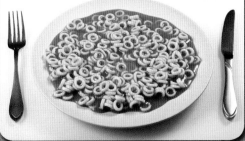

Weight: 420g (full tin)

Apple Chutney

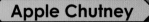

10g	38	0g	0g
CARBS	CALS	PROTEIN	FAT

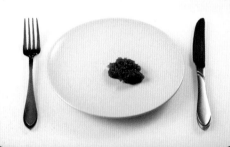

	CARBS	CALS	PROT	FAT
2x	20g	76	0g	0g
3x	30g	114	0g	0g
4x	40g	152	0g	0g
	Weight: 20g			

Brown Sauce

5g	21	0g	0g
CARBS	CALS	PROTEIN	FAT

	CARBS	CALS	PROT	FAT
2x	10g	42	0g	0g
3x	15g	63	0g	0g
4x	20g	84	0g	0g
	Weight: 21g			

Cranberry Sauce

6g	21	0g	0g
CARBS	CALS	PROTEIN	FAT

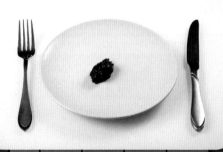

	CARBS	CALS	PROT	FAT
2x	12g	42	0g	0g
3x	18g	63	0g	0g
4x	24g	84	0g	0g
	Weight: 14g			

Horseradish

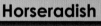

5g	40	1g	2g
CARBS	CALS	PROTEIN	FAT

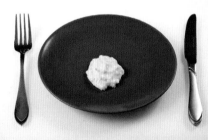

	CARBS	CALS	PROT	FAT
2x	10g	80	2g	4g
3x	15g	120	3g	6g
4x	20g	160	4g	8g
	Weight: 26g			

Ketchup

5g CARBS	22 CALS	0g PROTEIN	0g FAT

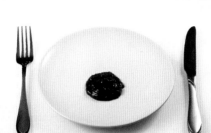

	CARBS	CALS	PROT	FAT
2x	10g	44	0g	0g
3x	15g	66	0g	0g
4x	20g	88	0g	0g

Weight: 19g

Mint Sauce

5g CARBS	21 CALS	0g PROTEIN	0g FAT

	CARBS	CALS	PROT	FAT
2x	10g	42	0g	0g
3x	15g	63	0g	0g
4x	20g	84	0g	0g

Weight: 21g

Piccalilli

4g CARBS	18 CALS	0g PROTEIN	0g FAT

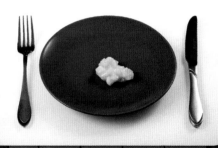

	CARBS	CALS	PROT	FAT
2x	8g	36	0g	0g
3x	12g	54	0g	0g
4x	16g	72	0g	0g

Weight: 22g

Pickle

10g CARBS	39 CALS	0g PROTEIN	0g FAT

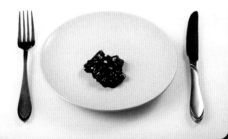

	CARBS	CALS	PROT	FAT
2x	20g	78	0g	0g
3x	30g	117	0g	0g
4x	40g	156	0g	0g

Weight: 28g

Salad Cream

5g	94	0g	8g
CARBS	CALS	PROTEIN	FAT

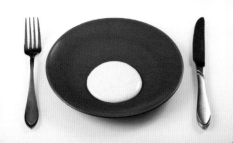

	CARBS	CALS	PROT	FAT
2x	10g	188	0g	16g
3x	15g	282	0g	24g
4x	20g	376	0g	32g
Weight: 27g			

Sweet Chilli Sauce

6g	23	0g	0g
CARBS	CALS	PROTEIN	FAT

	CARBS	CALS	PROT	FAT
2x	12g	46	0g	0g
3x	18g	69	0g	0g
4x	24g	92	0g	0g
Weight: 10g			

Tartar Sauce

5g	78	0g	6g
CARBS	CALS	PROTEIN	FAT

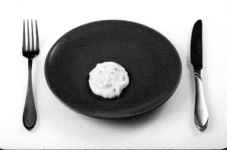

	CARBS	CALS	PROT	FAT
2x	10g	156	0g	12g
3x	15g	234	0g	18g
4x	20g	312	0g	24g
Weight: 26g			

Thousand Island

5g	116	0g	11g
CARBS	CALS	PROTEIN	FAT

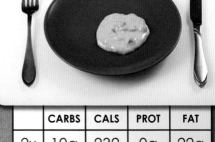

	CARBS	CALS	PROT	FAT
2x	10g	232	0g	22g
3x	15g	348	0g	33g
4x	20g	464	0g	44g
Weight: 36g			

Olive / Vegetable Oil

0g CARBS	36 CALS	0g PROTEIN	4g FAT

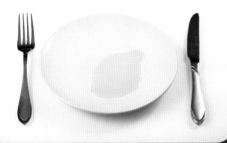

Weight: 4g (teaspoon)

Butter

0g CARBS	37 CALS	0g PROTEIN	4g FAT

Weight: 5g (teaspoon)

0g CARBS	99 CALS	0g PROTEIN	11g FAT

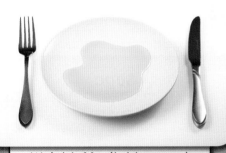

Weight: 11g (tablespoon)

0g CARBS	74 CALS	0g PROTEIN	8g FAT

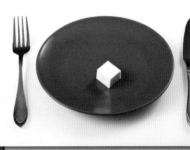

Weight: 10g

Mayonnaise

0g CARBS	104 CALS	0g PROTEIN	11g FAT

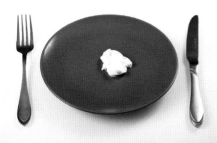

Weight: 15g

0g CARBS	112 CALS	0g PROTEIN	12g FAT

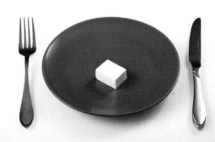

Weight: 15g

Honey

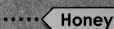

8g CARBS	29 CALS	0g PROTEIN	0g FAT

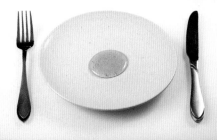

	CARBS	CALS	PROT	FAT
2x	16g	58	0g	0g
3x	24g	87	0g	0g
4x	32g	116	0g	0g
Weight: 10g (teaspoon)				

Jam

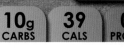

10g CARBS	39 CALS	0g PROTEIN	0g FAT

	CARBS	CALS	PROT	FAT
2x	20g	78	0g	0g
3x	30g	117	0g	0g
4x	40g	156	0g	0g
Weight: 15g (teaspoon)				

Marmalade

10g CARBS	39 CALS	0g PROTEIN	0g FAT

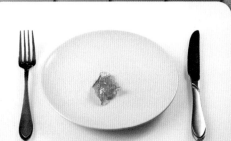

	CARBS	CALS	PROT	FAT
2x	20g	78	0g	0g
3x	30g	117	0g	0g
4x	40g	156	0g	0g
Weight: 15g (teaspoon)				

Sugar

5g CARBS	20 CALS	0g PROTEIN	0g FAT

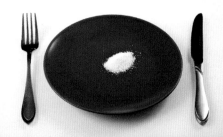

	CARBS	CALS	PROT	FAT
2x	10g	40	0g	0g
3x	15g	60	0g	0g
4x	20g	80	0g	0g
Weight: 5g (teaspoon)				

Chocolate Nut Spread

| 9g CARBS | 82 CALS | 1g PROTEIN | 5g FAT |

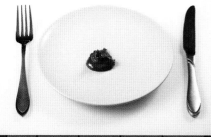

	CARBS	CALS	PROT	FAT
2x	18g	164	2g	10g
3x	27g	246	3g	15g
4x	36g	328	4g	20g
Weight: 15g				

Lemon Curd

| 9g CARBS | 42 CALS | 0g PROTEIN | 1g FAT |

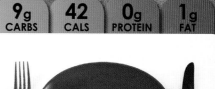

	CARBS	CALS	PROT	FAT
2x	18g	84	0g	2g
3x	27g	126	0g	3g
4x	36g	168	0g	4g
Weight: 15g				

Peanut Butter (crunchy)

| 2g CARBS | 91 CALS | 4g PROTEIN | 8g FAT |

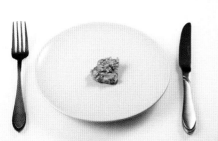

	CARBS	CALS	PROT	FAT
2x	4g	182	8g	16g
3x	6g	273	12g	24g
4x	8g	364	16g	32g
Weight: 15g				

Peanut Butter (smooth)

| 2g CARBS | 92 CALS | 4g PROTEIN | 8g FAT |

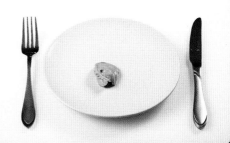

	CARBS	CALS	PROT	FAT
2x	4g	184	8g	16g
3x	6g	276	12g	24g
4x	8g	368	16g	32g
Weight: 15g				

Single Cream

| 0g CARBS | 15 CALS | 0g PROTEIN | 2g FAT |

| 0g CARBS | 31 CALS | 1g PROTEIN | 3g FAT |

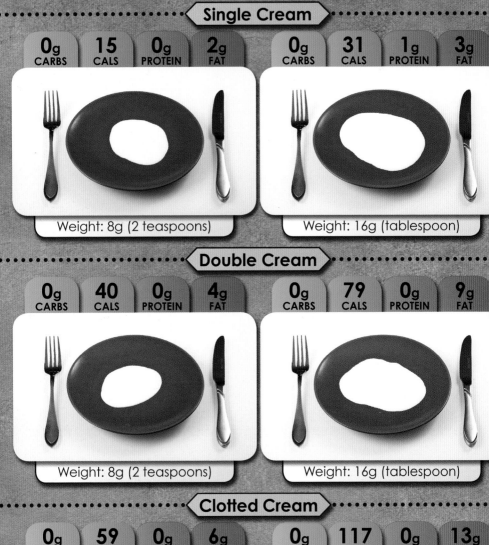

Weight: 8g (2 teaspoons)

Weight: 16g (tablespoon)

Double Cream

| 0g CARBS | 40 CALS | 0g PROTEIN | 4g FAT |

| 0g CARBS | 79 CALS | 0g PROTEIN | 9g FAT |

Weight: 8g (2 teaspoons)

Weight: 16g (tablespoon)

Clotted Cream

| 0g CARBS | 59 CALS | 0g PROTEIN | 6g FAT |

| 0g CARBS | 117 CALS | 0g PROTEIN | 13g FAT |

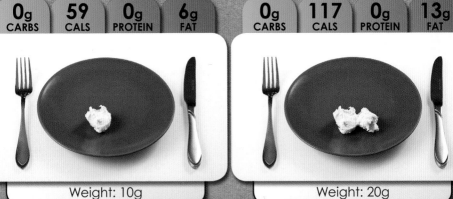

Weight: 10g

Weight: 20g

Crisps

10g CARBS	95 CALS	1g PROTEIN	6g FAT

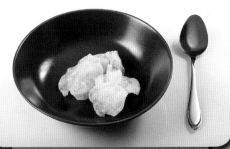

Weight: 18g

20g CARBS	201 CALS	2g PROTEIN	13g FAT

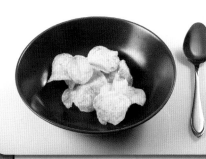

Weight: 38g

30g CARBS	297 CALS	3g PROTEIN	19g FAT

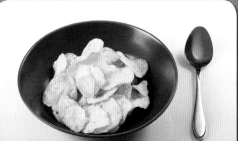

Weight: 56g

40g CARBS	398 CALS	4g PROTEIN	26g FAT

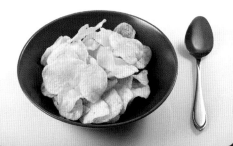

Weight: 75g

50g CARBS	498 CALS	5g PROTEIN	32g FAT

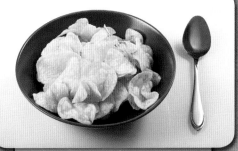

Weight: 94g

60g CARBS	594 CALS	6g PROTEIN	38g FAT

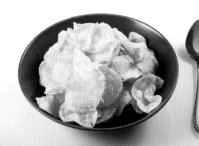

Weight: 112g

Bombay Mix

| 10g CARBS | 141 CALS | 5g PROTEIN | 9g FAT |

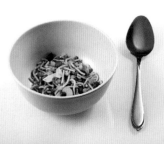

Weight: 28g

| 20g CARBS | 282 CALS | 11g PROTEIN | 18g FAT |

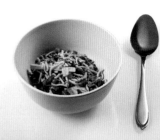

Weight: 56g

| 30g CARBS | 428 CALS | 16g PROTEIN | 28g FAT |

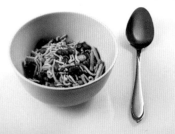

Weight: 85g

Cashew Nuts

| 5g CARBS | 171 CALS | 6g PROTEIN | 14g FAT |

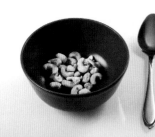

Weight: 28g

| 10g CARBS | 336 CALS | 11g PROTEIN | 28g FAT |

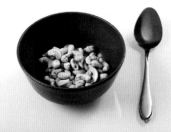

Weight: 55g

| 15g CARBS | 489 CALS | 16g PROTEIN | 41g FAT |

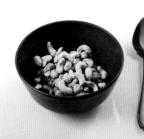

Weight: 80g

Dried Fruit & Nuts

10g CARBS	99 CALS	2g PROTEIN	5g FAT

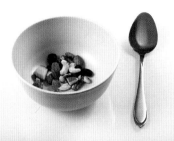

Weight: 22g

20g CARBS	198 CALS	5g PROTEIN	11g FAT

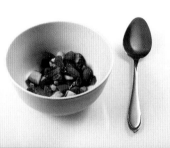

Weight: 44g

30g CARBS	297 CALS	7g PROTEIN	16g FAT

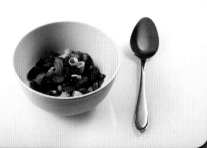

Weight: 66g

Peanuts (roasted)

5g CARBS	421 CALS	17g PROTEIN	37g FAT

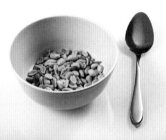

Weight: 70g

10g CARBS	843 CALS	34g PROTEIN	74g FAT

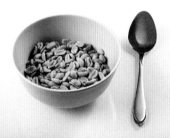

Weight: 140g

15g CARBS	1264 CALS	51g PROTEIN	111g FAT

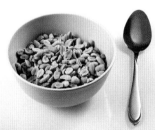

Weight: 210g

Popcorn (with butter)

5g CARBS	59 CALS	1g PROTEIN	4g FAT

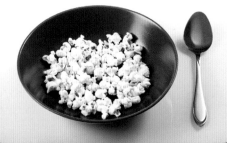

Weight: 10g

10g CARBS	119 CALS	1g PROTEIN	9g FAT

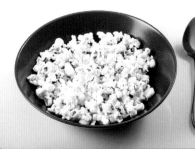

Weight: 20g

15g CARBS	178 CALS	2g PROTEIN	13g FAT

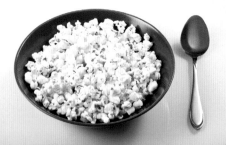

Weight: 30g

20g CARBS	243 CALS	3g PROTEIN	18g FAT

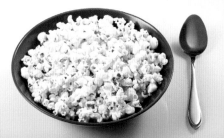

Weight: 41g

25g CARBS	302 CALS	3g PROTEIN	22g FAT

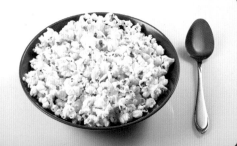

Weight: 51g

30g CARBS	362 CALS	4g PROTEIN	26g FAT

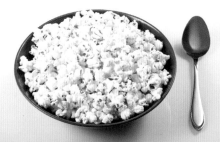

Weight: 61g

Popcorn (sweet)

17g CARBS	106 CALS	0g PROTEIN	4g FAT

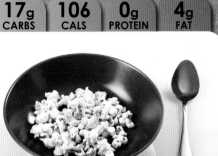

Weight: 22g

35g CARBS	216 CALS	1g PROTEIN	9g FAT

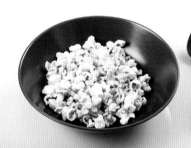

Weight: 45g

53g CARBS	326 CALS	1g PROTEIN	14g FAT

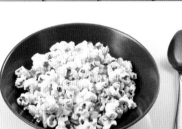

Weight: 68g

70g CARBS	432 CALS	2g PROTEIN	18g FAT

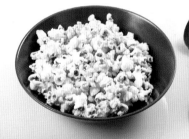

Weight: 90g

88g CARBS	542 CALS	2g PROTEIN	23g FAT

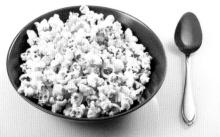

Weight: 113g

105g CARBS	648 CALS	3g PROTEIN	27g FAT

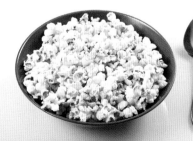

Weight: 135g

Prawn Crackers

5g CARBS	51 CALS	0g PROTEIN	4g FAT

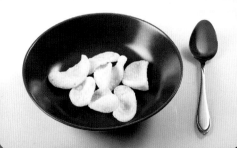

Weight: 9g

10g CARBS	103 CALS	0g PROTEIN	7g FAT

Weight: 18g

20g CARBS	200 CALS	0g PROTEIN	14g FAT

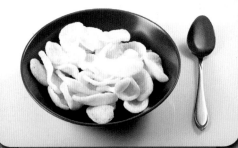

Weight: 35g

30g CARBS	296 CALS	0g PROTEIN	20g FAT

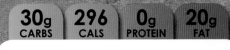

Weight: 52g

40g CARBS	388 CALS	0g PROTEIN	27g FAT

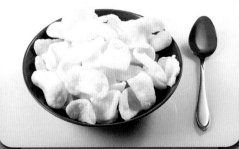

Weight: 68g

50g CARBS	490 CALS	0g PROTEIN	34g FAT

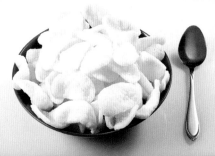

Weight: 86g

Tortilla Chips | Houmous

10g CARBS	30 CALS	1g PROTEIN	4g FAT

5g CARBS	84 CALS	3g PROTEIN	6g FAT

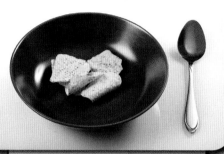 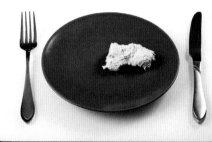

Weight: 16g | Weight: 45g

30g CARBS	230 CALS	4g PROTEIN	11g FAT

10g CARBS	168 CALS	7g PROTEIN	11g FAT

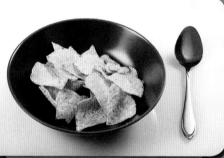 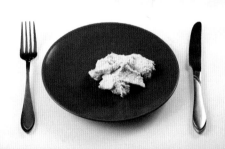

Weight: 50g | Weight: 90g

60g CARBS	459 CALS	8g PROTEIN	23g FAT

15g CARBS	243 CALS	10g PROTEIN	16g FAT

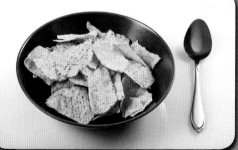 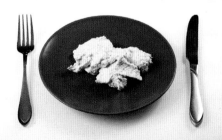

Weight: 100g | Weight: 130g

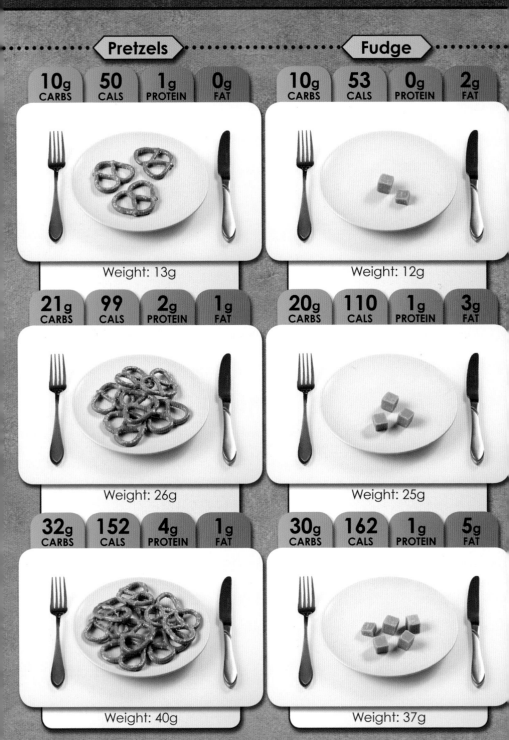

Pretzels

| 10g CARBS | 50 CALS | 1g PROTEIN | 0g FAT |

Weight: 13g

| 21g CARBS | 99 CALS | 2g PROTEIN | 1g FAT |

Weight: 26g

| 32g CARBS | 152 CALS | 4g PROTEIN | 1g FAT |

Weight: 40g

Fudge

| 10g CARBS | 53 CALS | 0g PROTEIN | 2g FAT |

Weight: 12g

| 20g CARBS | 110 CALS | 1g PROTEIN | 3g FAT |

Weight: 25g

| 30g CARBS | 162 CALS | 1g PROTEIN | 5g FAT |

Weight: 37g

Chocolate (milk)

9g CARBS	83 CALS	1g PROTEIN	5g FAT

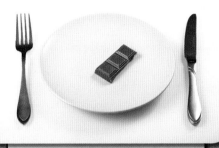

Weight: 16g

19g CARBS	172 CALS	3g PROTEIN	10g FAT

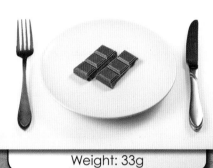

Weight: 33g

28g CARBS	260 CALS	4g PROTEIN	15g FAT

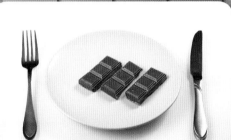

Weight: 50g

38g CARBS	348 CALS	5g PROTEIN	21g FAT

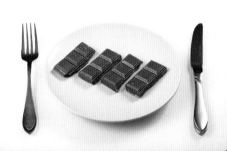

Weight: 67g

48g CARBS	442 CALS	7g PROTEIN	26g FAT

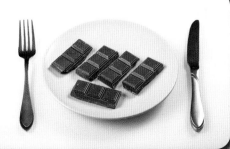

Weight: 85g

57g CARBS	525 CALS	8g PROTEIN	31g FAT

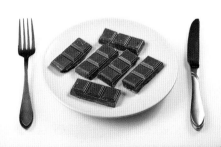

Weight: 101g

Chocolate (dark)

10g CARBS	82 CALS	1g PROTEIN	4g FAT

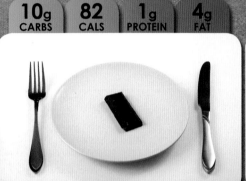

Weight: 16g

20g CARBS	163 CALS	2g PROTEIN	9g FAT

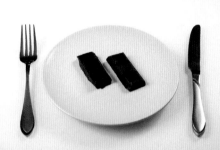

Weight: 32g

30g CARBS	245 CALS	2g PROTEIN	13g FAT

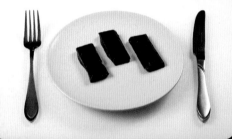

Weight: 48g

40g CARBS	321 CALS	3g PROTEIN	18g FAT

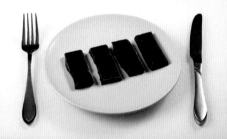

Weight: 63g

50g CARBS	398 CALS	4g PROTEIN	22g FAT

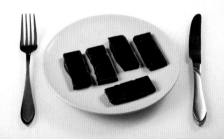

Weight: 78g

60g CARBS	479 CALS	5g PROTEIN	26g FAT

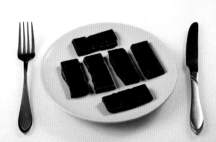

Weight: 94g

Chocolate Mint

9g CARBS	**70** CALS	**1**g PROTEIN	**3**g FAT

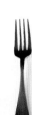
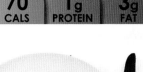
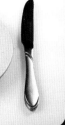

	CARBS	CALS	PROT	FAT
2x	18g	140	2g	6g
3x	27g	210	3g	9g
4x	36g	280	4g	12g
Weight: 15g				

Licorice Allsorts

9g CARBS	**42** CALS	**0**g PROTEIN	**1**g FAT

	CARBS	CALS	PROT	FAT
2x	18g	84	0g	2g
3x	27g	126	0g	3g
4x	36g	168	0g	4g
Weight: 12g				

Individual Chocolate

7g CARBS	**54** CALS	**1**g PROTEIN	**3**g FAT

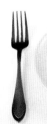
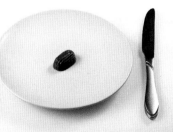

	CARBS	CALS	PROT	FAT
2x	14g	108	2g	6g
3x	21g	162	3g	9g
4x	28g	216	4g	12g
Weight: 11g				

8g CARBS	**71** CALS	**1**g PROTEIN	**4**g FAT

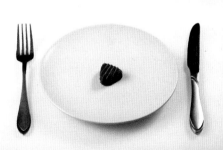

	CARBS	CALS	PROT	FAT
2x	16g	142	2g	8g
3x	24g	213	3g	12g
4x	32g	284	4g	16g
Weight: 14g				

Cola Bottles

10g CARBS	43 CALS	1g PROTEIN	0g FAT

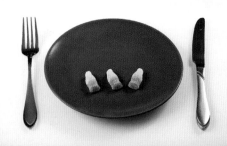

	CARBS	CALS	PROT	FAT
2x	20g	86	2g	0g
3x	30g	129	3g	0g
4x	40g	172	4g	0g
Weight: 13g				

Jelly Babies

15g CARBS	62 CALS	1g PROTEIN	0g FAT

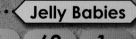

	CARBS	CALS	PROT	FAT
2x	30g	124	2g	0g
3x	45g	186	3g	0g
4x	60g	248	4g	0g
Weight: 18g				

Jelly Beans

10g CARBS	40 CALS	0g PROTEIN	0g FAT

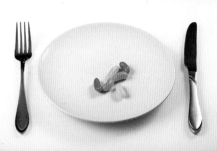

	CARBS	CALS	PROT	FAT
2x	20g	80	0g	0g
3x	30g	120	0g	0g
4x	40g	160	0g	0g
Weight: 11g				

Wine Gums

10g CARBS	45 CALS	1g PROTEIN	0g FAT

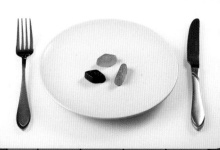

	CARBS	CALS	PROT	FAT
2x	20g	90	2g	0g
3x	30g	135	3g	0g
4x	40g	180	4g	0g
Weight: 14g				

Fish Stew with Jollof Rice

Fufu (yam)

46g CARBS	490 CALS	20g PROTEIN	26g FAT

49g CARBS	202 CALS	3g PROTEIN	0g FAT

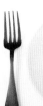
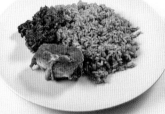
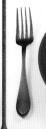

55g fish, 145g rice, 55g veg

Weight: 130g

96g CARBS	1024 CALS	42g PROTEIN	55g FAT

99g CARBS	411 CALS	6g PROTEIN	1g FAT

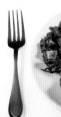
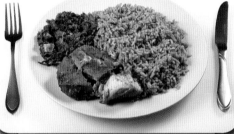
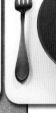
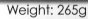

115g fish, 303g rice, 115g veg

Weight: 265g

142g CARBS	1513 CALS	62g PROTEIN	81g FAT

140g CARBS	581 CALS	8g PROTEIN	1g FAT

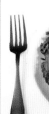
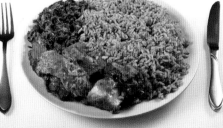
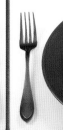

170g fish, 448g rice, 170g veg

Weight: 375g

Beef Burger (with cheese)

| 31g CARBS | 519 CALS | 37g PROTEIN | 29g FAT |

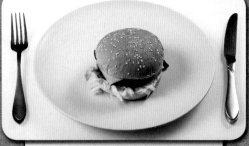

Weight: 181g

French Fries

| 33g CARBS | 269 CALS | 3g PROTEIN | 15g FAT |

Weight: 96g (small)

Chicken Burger

| 45g CARBS | 398 CALS | 24g PROTEIN | 15g FAT |

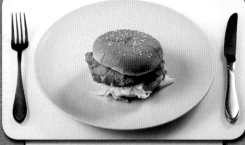

Weight: 168g

| 54g CARBS | 448 CALS | 5g PROTEIN | 25g FAT |

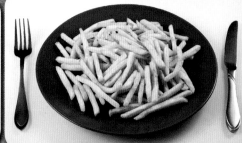

Weight: 160g (medium)

Veggie Burger

| 41g CARBS | 321 CALS | 15g PROTEIN | 12g FAT |

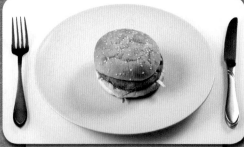

Weight: 158g

| 77g CARBS | 636 CALS | 7g PROTEIN | 35g FAT |

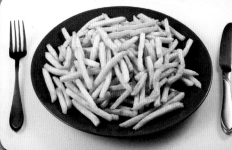

Weight: 227g (large)

Caribbean - Fried Fish, Rice & Peas

56g CARBS	555 CALS	24g PROTEIN	27g FAT

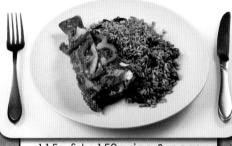

115g fish, 150g rice & peas

113g CARBS	1110 CALS	48g PROTEIN	55g FAT

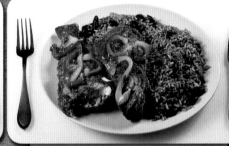

230g fish, 300g rice & peas

Caribbean - Goat & Potato Curry, Rice & Peas

76g CARBS	859 CALS	36g PROTEIN	51g FAT

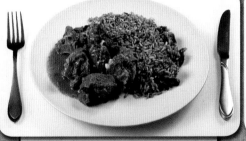

225g curry, 150g rice & peas

154g CARBS	1718 CALS	71g PROTEIN	101g FAT

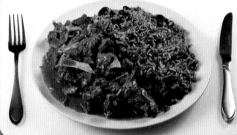

450g curry, 300g rice & peas

Caribbean - Jerk Chicken, Rice & Peas

49g CARBS	511 CALS	30g PROTEIN	22g FAT

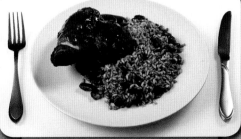

210g chicken, 150g rice & peas

98g CARBS	1023 CALS	62g PROTEIN	45g FAT

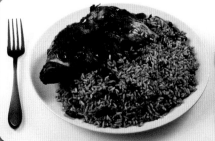

420g chicken, 300g rice & peas

Caribbean - Jamaican Beef Patty

27g CARBS	279 CALS	5g PROTEIN	17g FAT

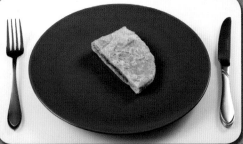

Weight: 85g

54g CARBS	551 CALS	11g PROTEIN	33g FAT

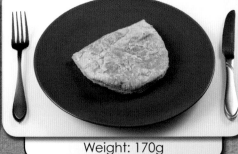

Weight: 170g

Caribbean - Rice & Peas

45g CARBS	240 CALS	8g PROTEIN	4g FAT

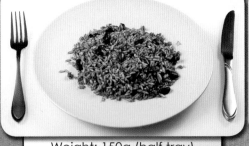

Weight: 150g (half tray)

91g CARBS	480 CALS	16g PROTEIN	8g FAT

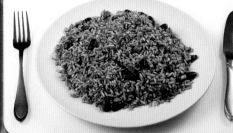

Weight: 300g (full tray)

Chinese - Duck Pancake

5g CARBS	106 CALS	5g PROTEIN	5g FAT

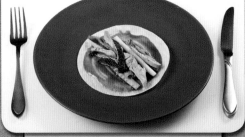

Weight: 50g

5g CARBS	106 CALS	5g PROTEIN	5g FAT

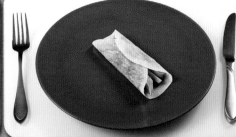

Weight: 50g

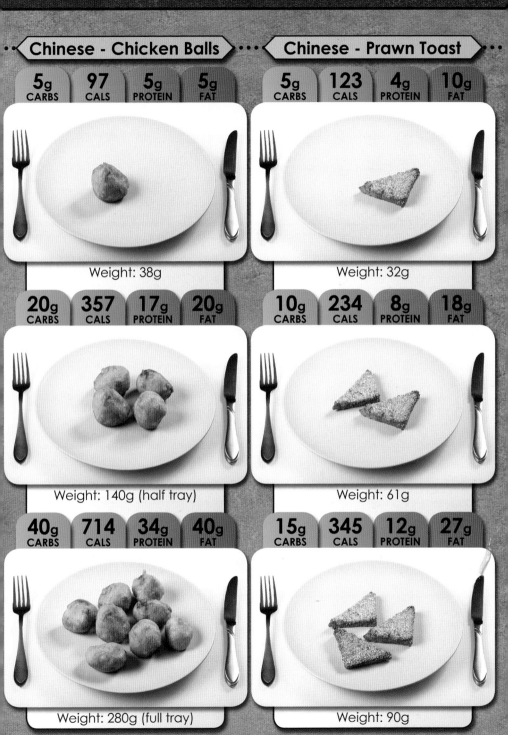

Chinese - Chicken Balls

5g CARBS	97 CALS	5g PROTEIN	5g FAT

Weight: 38g

20g CARBS	357 CALS	17g PROTEIN	20g FAT

Weight: 140g (half tray)

40g CARBS	714 CALS	34g PROTEIN	40g FAT

Weight: 280g (full tray)

Chinese - Prawn Toast

5g CARBS	123 CALS	4g PROTEIN	10g FAT

Weight: 32g

10g CARBS	234 CALS	8g PROTEIN	18g FAT

Weight: 61g

15g CARBS	345 CALS	12g PROTEIN	27g FAT

Weight: 90g

Chinese - Beef Chow Mein

40g CARBS	**374** CALS	**18**g PROTEIN	**17**g FAT

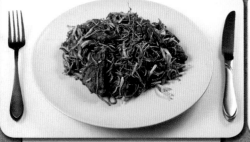

Weight: 275g (half tray)

80g CARBS	**741** CALS	**37**g PROTEIN	**33**g FAT

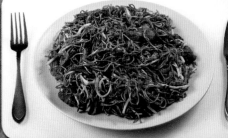

Weight: 545g (full tray)

Chinese - Chicken Curry

5g CARBS	**276** CALS	**22**g PROTEIN	**19**g FAT

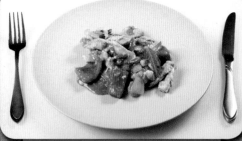

Weight: 190g (half tray)

10g CARBS	**551** CALS	**44**g PROTEIN	**37**g FAT

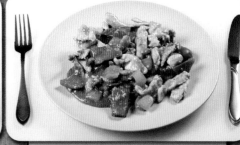

Weight: 380g (full tray)

Chinese - Singapore Noodles

26g CARBS	**223** CALS	**12**g PROTEIN	**8**g FAT

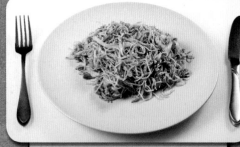

Weight: 205g (half tray)

52g CARBS	**447** CALS	**24**g PROTEIN	**16**g FAT

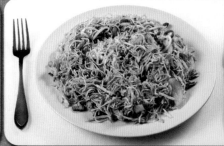

Weight: 410g (full tray)

Chinese - Egg Fried Rice

| **60g** CARBS | **335** CALS | **8g** PROTEIN | **9g** FAT | | **120g** CARBS | **670** CALS | **15g** PROTEIN | **18g** FAT |

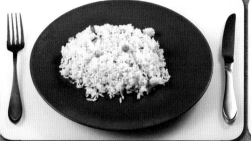
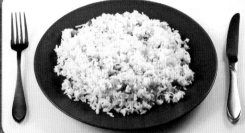

Weight: 180g (half tray)   Weight: 360g (full tray)

Chinese - Spring Roll

| **5g** CARBS | **52** CALS | **2g** PROTEIN | **3g** FAT | | **15g** CARBS | **152** CALS | **5g** PROTEIN | **9g** FAT |

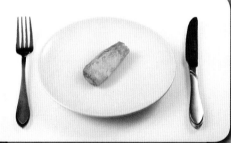
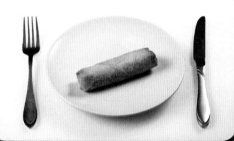

Weight: 24g   Weight: 70g

Chinese - Spare Ribs

| **15g** CARBS | **368** CALS | **27g** PROTEIN | **22g** FAT | | **31g** CARBS | **747** CALS | **55g** PROTEIN | **45g** FAT |

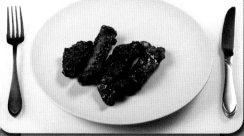
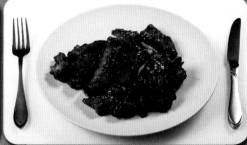

Weight: 150g (half tray)   Weight: 305g (full tray)

Chip Shop - Fish

16g CARBS	333 CALS	22g PROTEIN	21g FAT

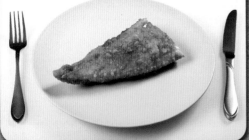

Weight: 135g

39g CARBS	815 CALS	53g PROTEIN	51g FAT

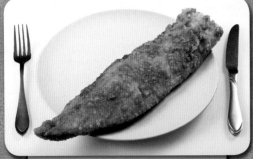

Weight: 330g

Chip Shop - Chips

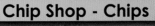

40g CARBS	311 CALS	4g PROTEIN	16g FAT

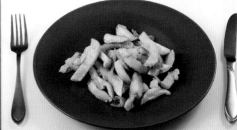

Weight: 130g

80g CARBS	626 CALS	8g PROTEIN	32g FAT

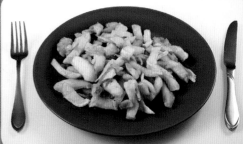

Weight: 262g

Battered Sausage

25g CARBS	421 CALS	16g PROTEIN	29g FAT

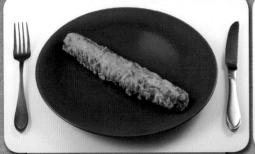

Weight: 137g

120g CARBS	944 CALS	13g PROTEIN	49g FAT

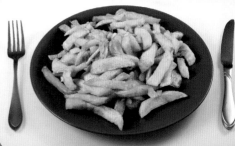

Weight: 395g

Indian - Onion Bhaji

15g CARBS	205 CALS	6g PROTEIN	14g FAT

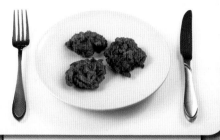

Weight: 66g

15g CARBS	205 CALS	6g PROTEIN	14g FAT

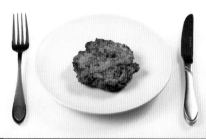

Weight: 66g

Indian - Pakora

5g CARBS	52 CALS	1g PROTEIN	3g FAT

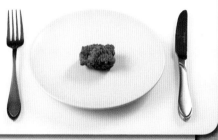

Weight: 22g

10g CARBS	106 CALS	3g PROTEIN	7g FAT

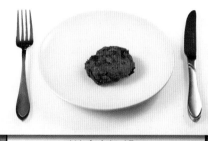

Weight: 45g

Indian - Samosa (meat)

6g CARBS	82 CALS	3g PROTEIN	6g FAT

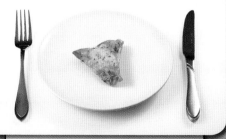

Weight: 30g

11g CARBS	158 CALS	7g PROTEIN	11g FAT

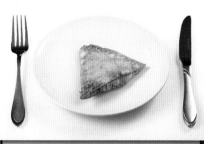

Weight: 58g

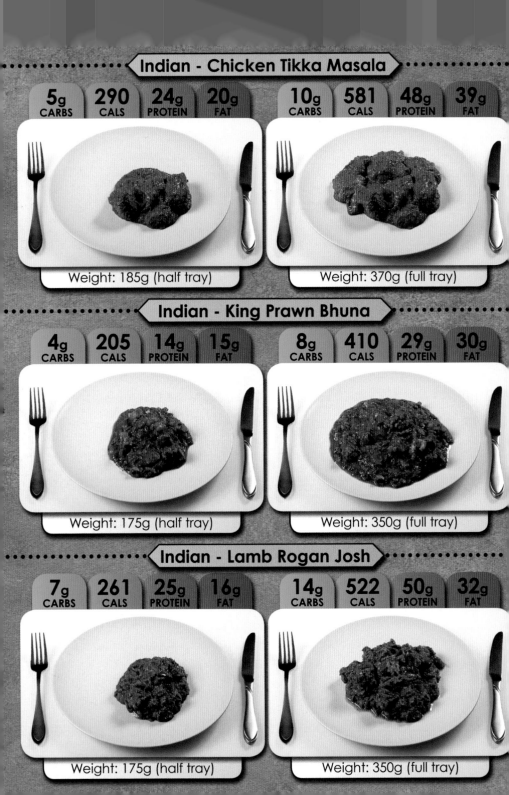

Indian - Chicken Tikka Masala

| 5g CARBS | 290 CALS | 24g PROTEIN | 20g FAT | | 10g CARBS | 581 CALS | 48g PROTEIN | 39g FAT |

Weight: 185g (half tray)

Weight: 370g (full tray)

Indian - King Prawn Bhuna

| 4g CARBS | 205 CALS | 14g PROTEIN | 15g FAT | | 8g CARBS | 410 CALS | 29g PROTEIN | 30g FAT |

Weight: 175g (half tray)

Weight: 350g (full tray)

Indian - Lamb Rogan Josh

| 7g CARBS | 261 CALS | 25g PROTEIN | 16g FAT | | 14g CARBS | 522 CALS | 50g PROTEIN | 32g FAT |

Weight: 175g (half tray)

Weight: 350g (full tray)

Indian - Bombay Potatoes

21g CARBS	177 CALS	3g PROTEIN	10g FAT

41g CARBS	354 CALS	6g PROTEIN	20g FAT

Weight: 150g (half tray)

Weight: 300g (full tray)

Indian - Sag Aloo Gobi

9g CARBS	124 CALS	3g PROTEIN	9g FAT

18g CARBS	247 CALS	6g PROTEIN	18g FAT

Weight: 130g (half tray)

Weight: 260g (full tray)

Indian - Sweet Mango Chutney

8g CARBS	30 CALS	0g PROTEIN	0g FAT

16g CARBS	62 CALS	0g PROTEIN	0g FAT

Weight: 16g

Weight: 33g

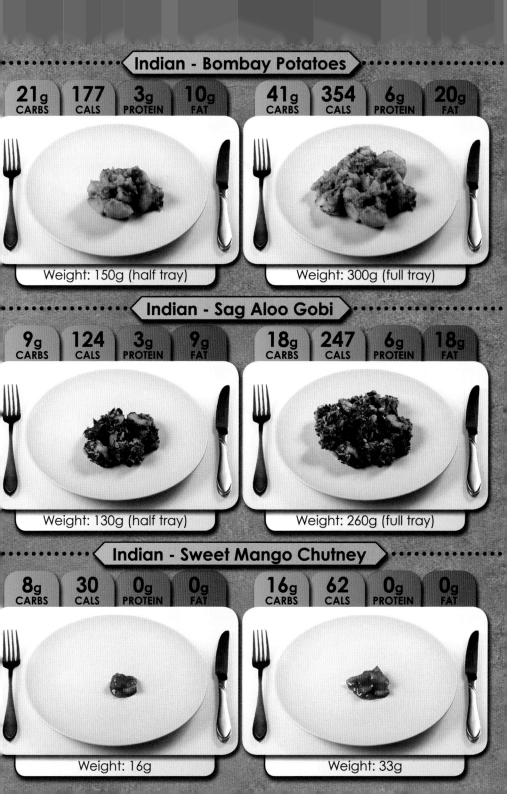

Doner Kebab

50g CARBS	580 CALS	29g PROTEIN	32g FAT

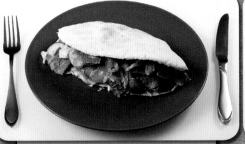

Weight: 250g (small)

80g CARBS	1053 CALS	53g PROTEIN	60g FAT

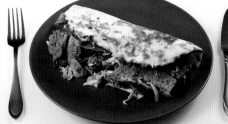

Weight: 415g (large)

Shish Kebab

50g CARBS	435 CALS	34g PROTEIN	14g FAT

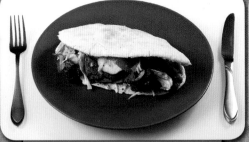

Weight: 250g (small)

80g CARBS	762 CALS	62g PROTEIN	24g FAT

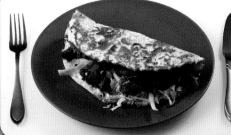

Weight: 415g (large)

Falafel in Pitta

60g CARBS	372 CALS	13g PROTEIN	11g FAT

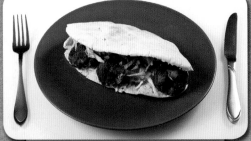

Weight: 200g (small)

100g CARBS	647 CALS	22g PROTEIN	21g FAT

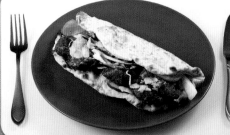

Weight: 350g (large)

Pizza (meat, deep pan)

21g CARBS	176 CALS	9g PROTEIN	7g FAT

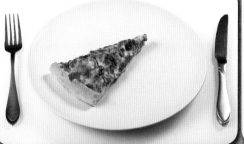

	CARBS	CALS	PROT	FAT
2x	42g	352	18g	14g
3x	63g	528	27g	21g
4x	84g	704	36g	28g
Weight: 70g				

41g CARBS	353 CALS	18g PROTEIN	14g FAT

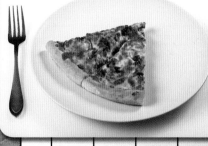

	CARBS	CALS	PROT	FAT
2x	82g	706	36g	28g
3x	123g	1059	54g	42g
4x	164g	1412	72g	56g
Weight: 140g				

62g CARBS	524 CALS	27g PROTEIN	20g FAT

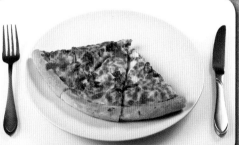

	CARBS	CALS	PROT	FAT
2x	124g	1048	54g	40g
3x	186g	1572	81g	60g
4x	248g	2096	108g	80g
Weight: 208g				

82g CARBS	698 CALS	35g PROTEIN	27g FAT

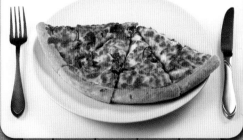

	CARBS	CALS	PROT	FAT
2x	164g	1396	70g	54g
3x	246g	2094	105g	81g
4x	328g	2792	140g	108g
Weight: 277g				

Pizza (vegetable, thin crust)

13g CARBS	**126** CALS	**6g** PROTEIN	**6g** FAT

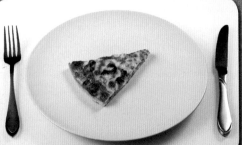

	CARBS	CALS	PROT	FAT
2x	26g	252	12g	12g
3x	39g	378	18g	18g
4x	52g	504	24g	24g
Weight: 50g				

26g CARBS	**252** CALS	**12g** PROTEIN	**11g** FAT

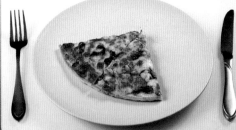

	CARBS	CALS	PROT	FAT
2x	52g	504	24g	22g
3x	78g	756	36g	33g
4x	104g	1008	48g	44g
Weight: 100g				

39g CARBS	**378** CALS	**18g** PROTEIN	**17g** FAT

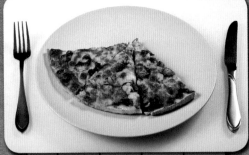

	CARBS	CALS	PROT	FAT
2x	78g	756	36g	34g
3x	117g	1134	54g	51g
4x	156g	1512	72g	68g
Weight: 150g				

52g CARBS	**504** CALS	**24g** PROTEIN	**22g** FAT

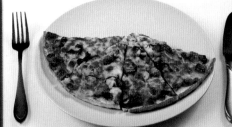

	CARBS	CALS	PROT	FAT
2x	104g	1008	48g	44g
3x	156g	1512	72g	66g
4x	208g	2016	96g	88g
Weight: 200g				

Pizza (pepperoni, stuffed crust)

20g CARBS	170 CALS	9g PROTEIN	7g FAT

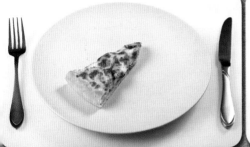

	CARBS	CALS	PROT	FAT
2x	40g	340	18g	14g
3x	60g	510	27g	21g
4x	80g	680	36g	28g
Weight: 65g				

40g CARBS	339 CALS	17g PROTEIN	15g FAT

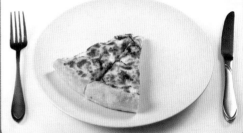

	CARBS	CALS	PROT	FAT
2x	80g	678	34g	30g
3x	120g	1017	51g	45g
4x	160g	1356	68g	60g
Weight: 130g				

60g CARBS	517 CALS	26g PROTEIN	22g FAT

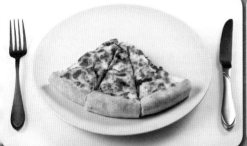

	CARBS	CALS	PROT	FAT
2x	120g	1034	52g	44g
3x	180g	1551	78g	66g
4x	240g	2068	104g	88g
Weight: 198g				

80g CARBS	684 CALS	34g PROTEIN	30g FAT

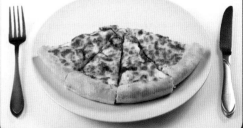

	CARBS	CALS	PROT	FAT
2x	160g	1368	68g	60g
3x	240g	2052	102g	90g
4x	320g	2736	136g	120g
Weight: 262g				

Thai - Green Curry

| 7g CARBS | 271 CALS | 29g PROTEIN | 14g FAT | 13g CARBS | 542 CALS | 58g PROTEIN | 29g FAT |

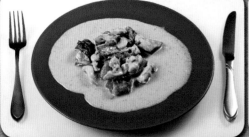 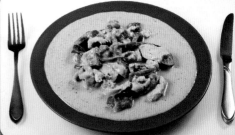

Weight: 195g (half tray)   Weight: 390g (full tray)

Thai - Phad Thai

| 49g CARBS | 325 CALS | 14g PROTEIN | 8g FAT | 97g CARBS | 649 CALS | 29g PROTEIN | 17g FAT |

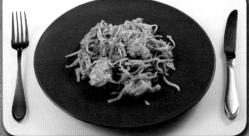 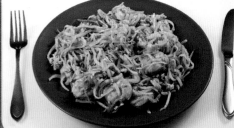

Weight: 200g (half tray)   Weight: 400g (full tray)

Thai - Pineapple, Chicken & Prawn Rice

| 69g CARBS | 483 CALS | 15g PROTEIN | 16g FAT | 139g CARBS | 965 CALS | 30g PROTEIN | 32g FAT |

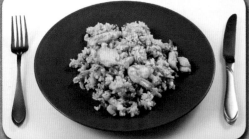 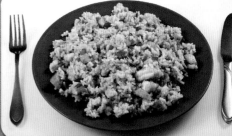

Weight: 250g (half tray)   Weight: 500g (full tray)

Asparagus (boiled)

1g CARBS	10 CALS	1g PROTEIN	0g FAT

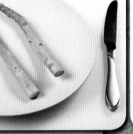

Weight: 40g

1g CARBS	21 CALS	3g PROTEIN	1g FAT

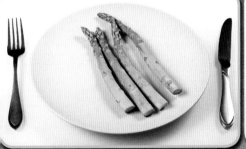

Weight: 80g

2g CARBS	31 CALS	4g PROTEIN	1g FAT

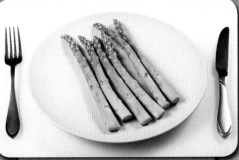

Weight: 120g

Aubergine (fried)

1g CARBS	91 CALS	0g PROTEIN	10g FAT

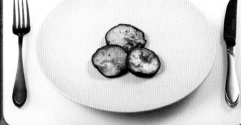

Weight: 30g

2g CARBS	181 CALS	1g PROTEIN	19g FAT

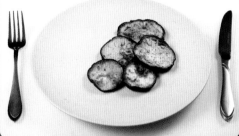

Weight: 60g

3g CARBS	272 CALS	1g PROTEIN	29g FAT

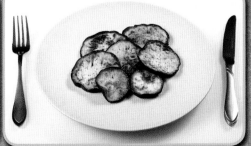

Weight: 90g

Avocado

| 1g CARBS | 67 CALS | 1g PROTEIN | 7g FAT |

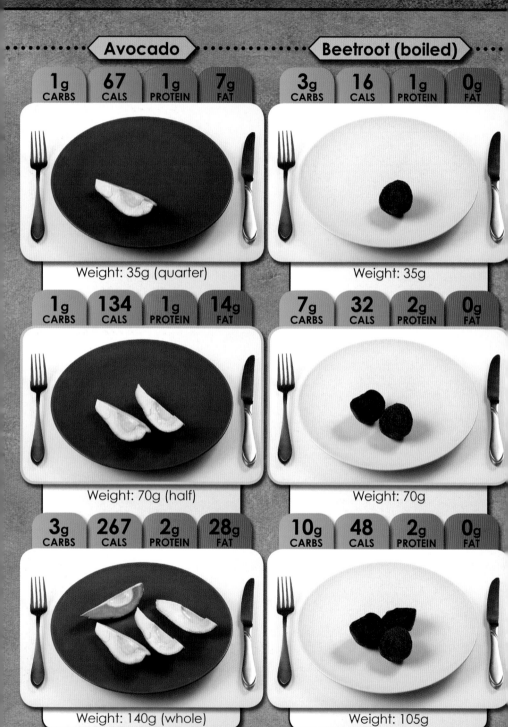

Weight: 35g (quarter)

| 1g CARBS | 134 CALS | 1g PROTEIN | 14g FAT |

Weight: 70g (half)

| 3g CARBS | 267 CALS | 2g PROTEIN | 28g FAT |

Weight: 140g (whole)

Beetroot (boiled)

| 3g CARBS | 16 CALS | 1g PROTEIN | 0g FAT |

Weight: 35g

| 7g CARBS | 32 CALS | 2g PROTEIN | 0g FAT |

Weight: 70g

| 10g CARBS | 48 CALS | 2g PROTEIN | 0g FAT |

Weight: 105g

Baked Beans

10g CARBS	**55** CALS	**3g** PROTEIN	**0g** FAT

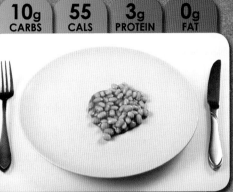

Weight: 65g

20g CARBS	**109** CALS	**7g** PROTEIN	**1g** FAT

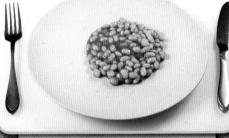

Weight: 130g

30g CARBS	**164** CALS	**10g** PROTEIN	**1g** FAT

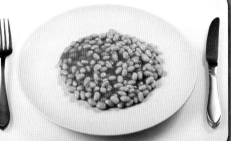

Weight: 195g (half tin)

40g CARBS	**218** CALS	**14g** PROTEIN	**2g** FAT

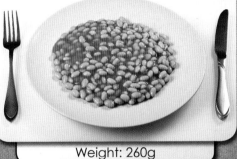

Weight: 260g

50g CARBS	**273** CALS	**17g** PROTEIN	**2g** FAT

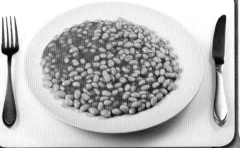

Weight: 325g

60g CARBS	**328** CALS	**20g** PROTEIN	**2g** FAT

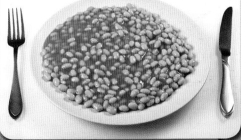

Weight: 390g (full tin)

Broad Beans (boiled)

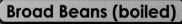

2g CARBS	14 CALS	2g PROTEIN	0g FAT

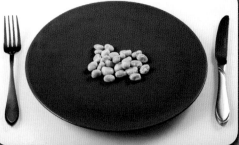

Weight: 30g

3g CARBS	29 CALS	3g PROTEIN	0g FAT

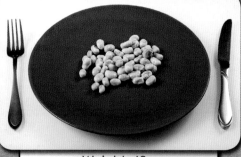

Weight: 60g

5g CARBS	43 CALS	5g PROTEIN	1g FAT

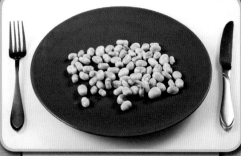

Weight: 90g

Green Beans (boiled)

1g CARBS	9 CALS	1g PROTEIN	0g FAT

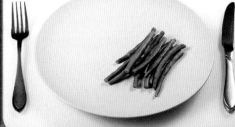

Weight: 40g

2g CARBS	18 CALS	1g PROTEIN	0g FAT

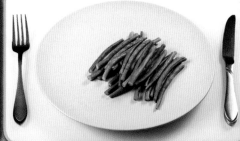

Weight: 80g

3g CARBS	26 CALS	2g PROTEIN	1g FAT

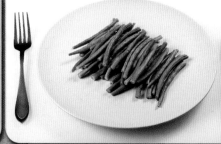

Weight: 120g

Kidney Beans

| 5g CARBS | 30 CALS | 2g PROTEIN | 0g FAT |

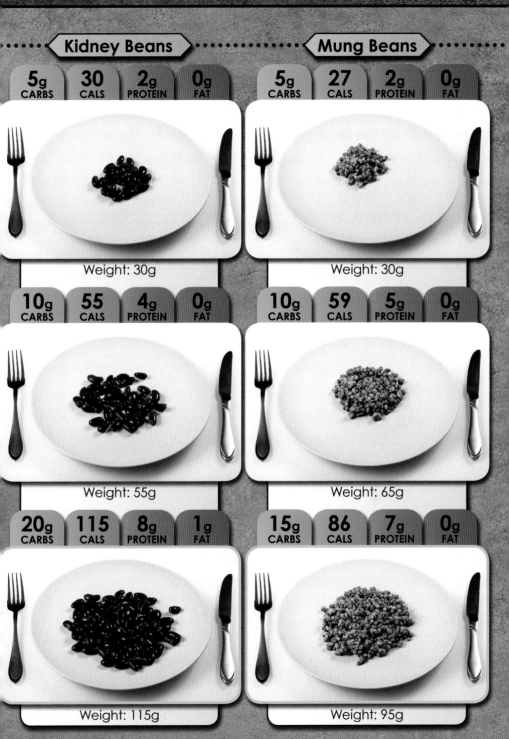

Weight: 30g

| 10g CARBS | 55 CALS | 4g PROTEIN | 0g FAT |

Weight: 55g

| 20g CARBS | 115 CALS | 8g PROTEIN | 1g FAT |

Weight: 115g

Mung Beans

| 5g CARBS | 27 CALS | 2g PROTEIN | 0g FAT |

Weight: 30g

| 10g CARBS | 59 CALS | 5g PROTEIN | 0g FAT |

Weight: 65g

| 15g CARBS | 86 CALS | 7g PROTEIN | 0g FAT |

Weight: 95g

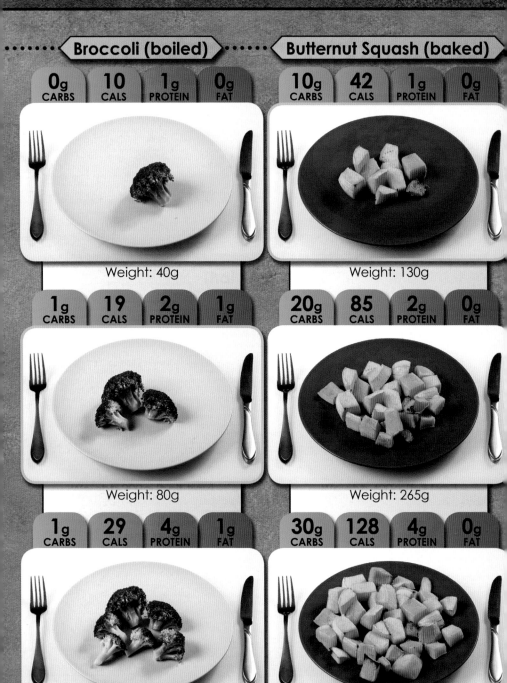

Broccoli (boiled)

0g CARBS | **10** CALS | **1g** PROTEIN | **0g** FAT

Weight: 40g

1g CARBS | **19** CALS | **2g** PROTEIN | **1g** FAT

Weight: 80g

1g CARBS | **29** CALS | **4g** PROTEIN | **1g** FAT

Weight: 120g

Butternut Squash (baked)

10g CARBS | **42** CALS | **1g** PROTEIN | **0g** FAT

Weight: 130g

20g CARBS | **85** CALS | **2g** PROTEIN | **0g** FAT

Weight: 265g

30g CARBS | **128** CALS | **4g** PROTEIN | **0g** FAT

Weight: 400g

Cabbage (boiled)

| 1g CARBS | 6 CALS | 0g PROTEIN | 0g FAT |

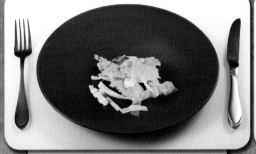

Weight: 40g

| 2g CARBS | 13 CALS | 1g PROTEIN | 0g FAT |

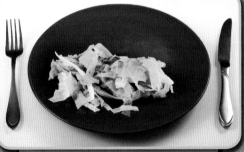

Weight: 80g

| 3g CARBS | 19 CALS | 1g PROTEIN | 0g FAT |

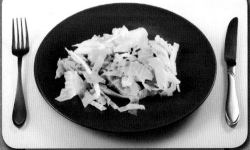

Weight: 120g

Carrots (boiled)

| 2g CARBS | 10 CALS | 0g PROTEIN | 0g FAT |

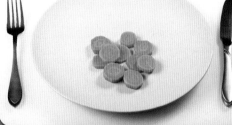

Weight: 40g

| 4g CARBS | 19 CALS | 0g PROTEIN | 0g FAT |

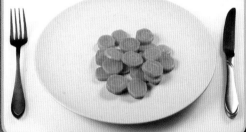

Weight: 80g

| 6g CARBS | 29 CALS | 1g PROTEIN | 0g FAT |

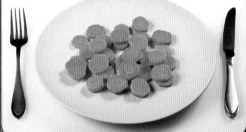

Weight: 120g

Cauliflower (boiled)

1g CARBS	11 CALS	1g PROTEIN	0g FAT

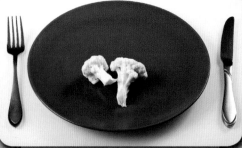

Weight: 40g

2g CARBS	22 CALS	2g PROTEIN	1g FAT

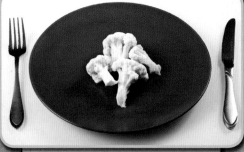

Weight: 80g

3g CARBS	34 CALS	3g PROTEIN	1g FAT

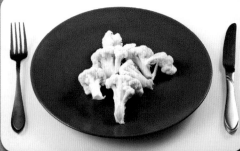

Weight: 120g

Celery

0g CARBS	2 CALS	0g PROTEIN	0g FAT

Weight: 30g

0g CARBS	2 CALS	0g PROTEIN	0g FAT

Weight: 30g

1g CARBS	4 CALS	0g PROTEIN	0g FAT

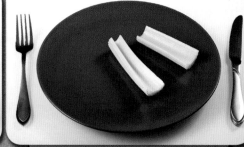

Weight: 60g

Cherry Tomatoes

1g CARBS	7 CALS	0g PROTEIN	0g FAT

Weight: 40g

2g CARBS	14 CALS	1g PROTEIN	0g FAT

Weight: 80g

4g CARBS	22 CALS	1g PROTEIN	0g FAT

Weight: 120g

Chick Peas

5g CARBS	35 CALS	2g PROTEIN	1g FAT

Weight: 30g

10g CARBS	69 CALS	4g PROTEIN	2g FAT

Weight: 60g

20g CARBS	144 CALS	9g PROTEIN	4g FAT

Weight: 125g

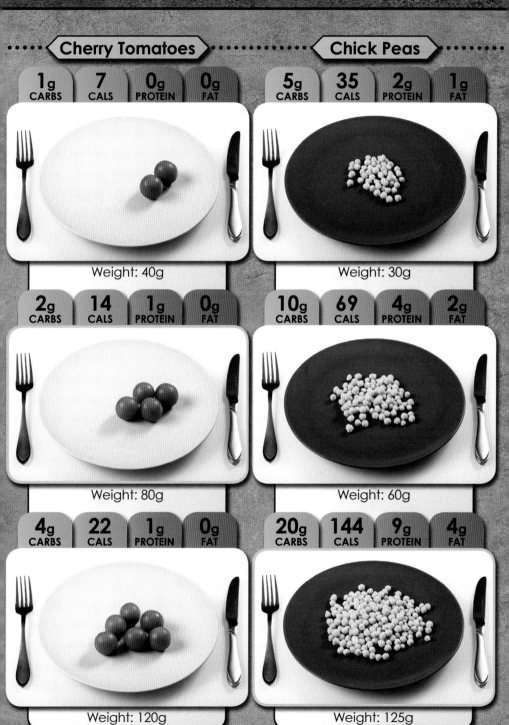

Courgette (boiled)

1g CARBS	8 CALS	1g PROTEIN	0g FAT

Weight: 40g

2g CARBS	15 CALS	2g PROTEIN	0g FAT

Weight: 80g

2g CARBS	23 CALS	2g PROTEIN	0g FAT

Weight: 120g

Cucumber

0g CARBS	2 CALS	0g PROTEIN	0g FAT

Weight: 22g

1g CARBS	4 CALS	0g PROTEIN	0g FAT

Weight: 44g

1g CARBS	7 CALS	0g PROTEIN	0g FAT

Weight: 66g

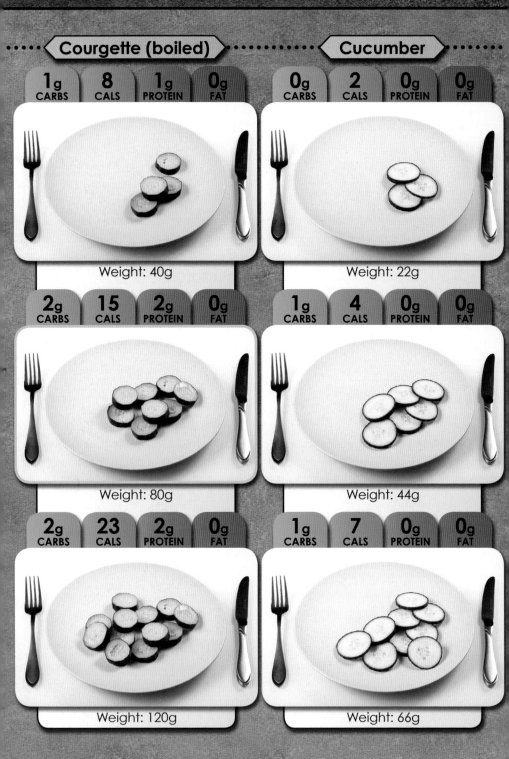

Leek (boiled)

1g CARBS	11 CALS	1g PROTEIN	0g FAT

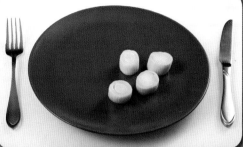

Weight: 50g

3g CARBS	21 CALS	1g PROTEIN	1g FAT

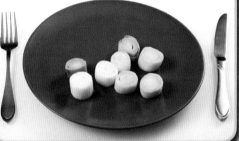

Weight: 100g

4g CARBS	32 CALS	2g PROTEIN	1g FAT

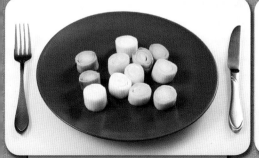

Weight: 150g

Lentils

10g CARBS	63 CALS	5g PROTEIN	0g FAT

Weight: 60g

20g CARBS	126 CALS	11g PROTEIN	1g FAT

Weight: 120g

30g CARBS	189 CALS	16g PROTEIN	1g FAT

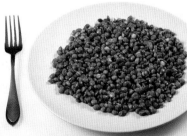

Weight: 180g

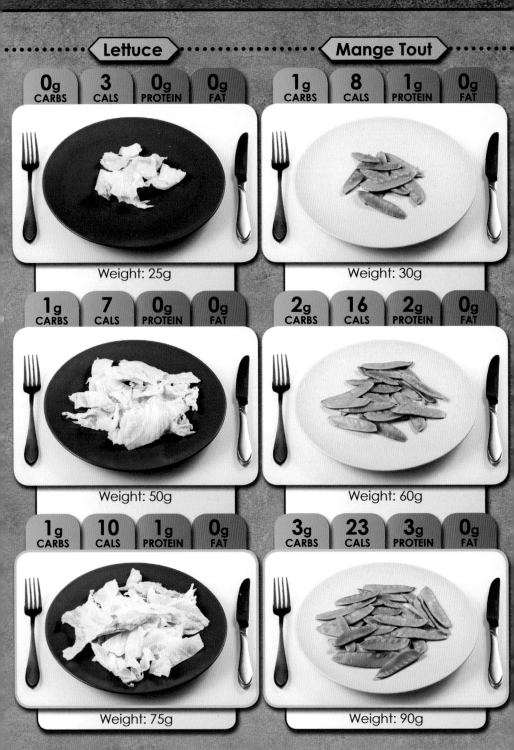

Lettuce

| 0g CARBS | 3 CALS | 0g PROTEIN | 0g FAT |

Weight: 25g

| 1g CARBS | 7 CALS | 0g PROTEIN | 0g FAT |

Weight: 50g

| 1g CARBS | 10 CALS | 1g PROTEIN | 0g FAT |

Weight: 75g

Mange Tout

| 1g CARBS | 8 CALS | 1g PROTEIN | 0g FAT |

Weight: 30g

| 2g CARBS | 16 CALS | 2g PROTEIN | 0g FAT |

Weight: 60g

| 3g CARBS | 23 CALS | 3g PROTEIN | 0g FAT |

Weight: 90g

Mushrooms (fried)

0g CARBS	63 CALS	1g PROTEIN	6g FAT

Weight: 40g

0g CARBS	126 CALS	2g PROTEIN	13g FAT

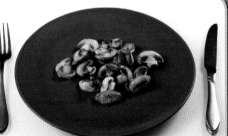

Weight: 80g

0g CARBS	188 CALS	3g PROTEIN	19g FAT

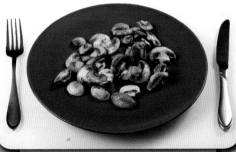

Weight: 120g

Okra (boiled)

1g CARBS	11 CALS	1g PROTEIN	0g FAT

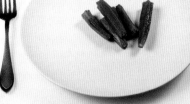

Weight: 40g

2g CARBS	22 CALS	2g PROTEIN	1g FAT

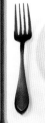

Weight: 80g

3g CARBS	34 CALS	3g PROTEIN	1g FAT

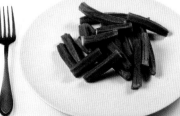

Weight: 120g

Onions (fried)

4g CARBS	49 CALS	1g PROTEIN	3g FAT

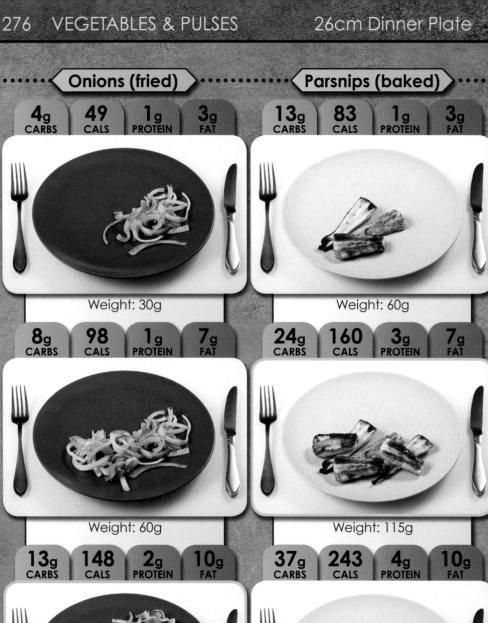

Weight: 30g

8g CARBS	98 CALS	1g PROTEIN	7g FAT

Weight: 60g

13g CARBS	148 CALS	2g PROTEIN	10g FAT

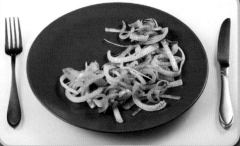

Weight: 90g

Parsnips (baked)

13g CARBS	83 CALS	1g PROTEIN	3g FAT

Weight: 60g

24g CARBS	160 CALS	3g PROTEIN	7g FAT

Weight: 115g

37g CARBS	243 CALS	4g PROTEIN	10g FAT

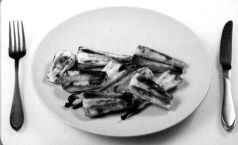

Weight: 175g

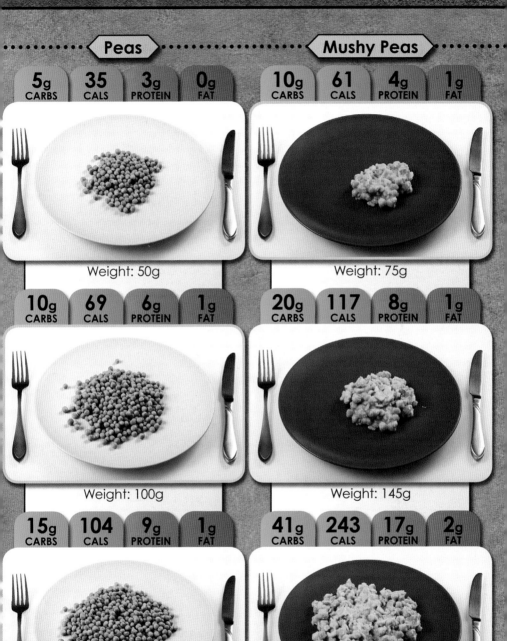

Peas

5g CARBS   **35** CALS   **3g** PROTEIN   **0g** FAT

Weight: 50g

Mushy Peas

10g CARBS   **61** CALS   **4g** PROTEIN   **1g** FAT

Weight: 75g

10g CARBS   **69** CALS   **6g** PROTEIN   **1g** FAT

Weight: 100g

20g CARBS   **117** CALS   **8g** PROTEIN   **1g** FAT

Weight: 145g

15g CARBS   **104** CALS   **9g** PROTEIN   **1g** FAT

Weight: 150g

41g CARBS   **243** CALS   **17g** PROTEIN   **2g** FAT

Weight: 300g

Peppers

| 1g CARBS | 5 CALS | 0g PROTEIN | 0g FAT |

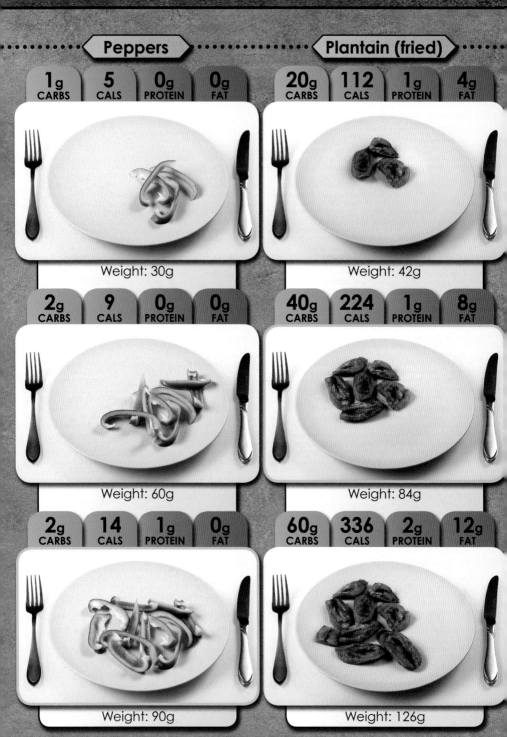

Weight: 30g

| 2g CARBS | 9 CALS | 0g PROTEIN | 0g FAT |

Weight: 60g

| 2g CARBS | 14 CALS | 1g PROTEIN | 0g FAT |

Weight: 90g

Plantain (fried)

| 20g CARBS | 112 CALS | 1g PROTEIN | 4g FAT |

Weight: 42g

| 40g CARBS | 224 CALS | 1g PROTEIN | 8g FAT |

Weight: 84g

| 60g CARBS | 336 CALS | 2g PROTEIN | 12g FAT |

Weight: 126g

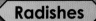

Radishes

0g CARBS	1 CALS	0g PROTEIN	0g FAT

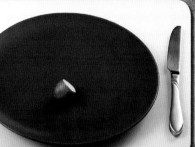

Weight: 12g

0g CARBS	3 CALS	0g PROTEIN	0g FAT

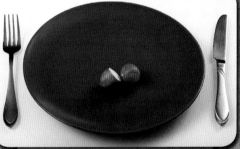

Weight: 24g

1g CARBS	4 CALS	0g PROTEIN	0g FAT

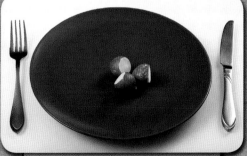

Weight: 36g

Salad Leaves

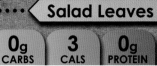

0g CARBS	3 CALS	0g PROTEIN	0g FAT

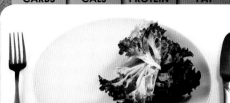

Weight: 20g

1g CARBS	6 CALS	0g PROTEIN	0g FAT

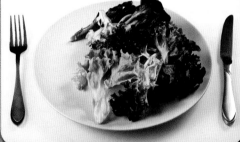

Weight: 40g

1g CARBS	8 CALS	0g PROTEIN	0g FAT

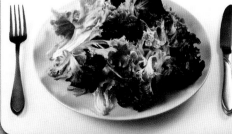

Weight: 60g

Spinach (boiled)

| 0g CARBS | 8 CALS | 1g PROTEIN | 0g FAT |

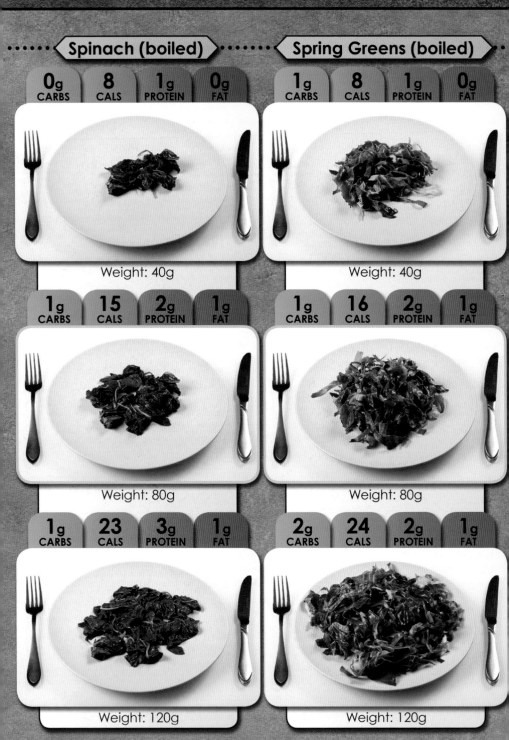

Weight: 40g

| 1g CARBS | 15 CALS | 2g PROTEIN | 1g FAT |

Weight: 80g

| 1g CARBS | 23 CALS | 3g PROTEIN | 1g FAT |

Weight: 120g

Spring Greens (boiled)

| 1g CARBS | 8 CALS | 1g PROTEIN | 0g FAT |

Weight: 40g

| 1g CARBS | 16 CALS | 2g PROTEIN | 1g FAT |

Weight: 80g

| 2g CARBS | 24 CALS | 2g PROTEIN | 1g FAT |

Weight: 120g

Sprouts (boiled)

2g CARBS	18 CALS	1g PROTEIN	1g FAT

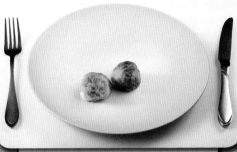

Weight: 50g

4g CARBS	35 CALS	3g PROTEIN	1g FAT

Weight: 100g

5g CARBS	53 CALS	4g PROTEIN	2g FAT

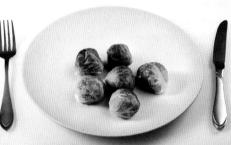

Weight: 150g

Sugar Snap Peas (boiled)

2g CARBS	13 CALS	1g PROTEIN	0g FAT

Weight: 40g

4g CARBS	26 CALS	2g PROTEIN	0g FAT

Weight: 80g

6g CARBS	40 CALS	4g PROTEIN	0g FAT

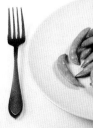

Weight: 120g

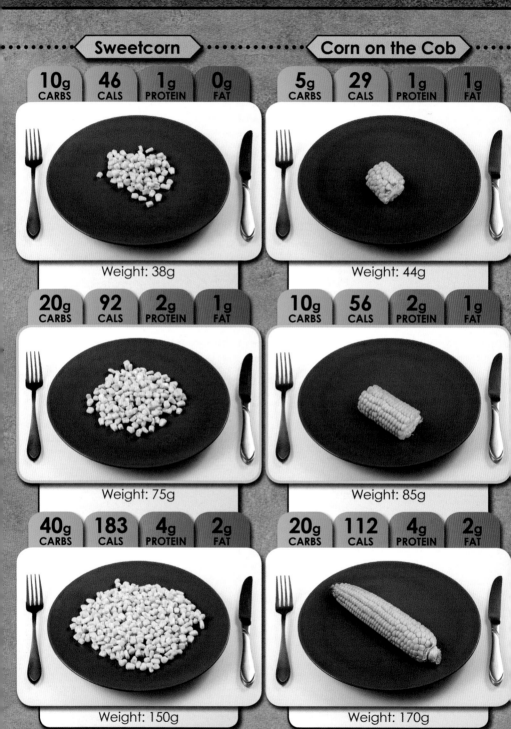

Sweetcorn

| 10g CARBS | 46 CALS | 1g PROTEIN | 0g FAT |

Weight: 38g

| 20g CARBS | 92 CALS | 2g PROTEIN | 1g FAT |

Weight: 75g

| 40g CARBS | 183 CALS | 4g PROTEIN | 2g FAT |

Weight: 150g

Corn on the Cob

| 5g CARBS | 29 CALS | 1g PROTEIN | 1g FAT |

Weight: 44g

| 10g CARBS | 56 CALS | 2g PROTEIN | 1g FAT |

Weight: 85g

| 20g CARBS | 112 CALS | 4g PROTEIN | 2g FAT |

Weight: 170g

Tomato

2g CARBS	9 CALS	0g PROTEIN	0g FAT

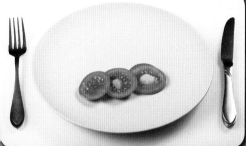

Weight: 50g (half)

2g CARBS	9 CALS	0g PROTEIN	0g FAT

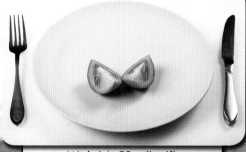

Weight: 50g (half)

4g CARBS	20 CALS	1g PROTEIN	0g FAT

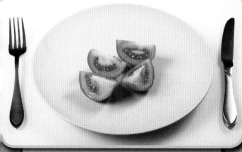

Weight: 115g (whole)

Yam (boiled)

20g CARBS	80 CALS	1g PROTEIN	0g FAT

Weight: 60g

40g CARBS	160 CALS	2g PROTEIN	0g FAT

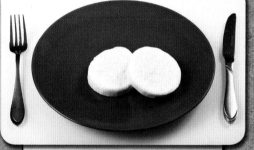

Weight: 120g

60g CARBS	242 CALS	3g PROTEIN	1g FAT

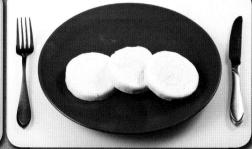

Weight: 182g

Index

Acknowledgements

We hope that you have enjoyed this book and continue to find it useful for years to come. It has been great fun producing the final product and we hope it helps thousands of people to understand the carbohydrate, calorie, protein and fat content of the food they eat.

We would like to take the opportunity to express our deepest thanks and appreciation to the two most special people in our lives - Justine and Chrissi.

We would also like to thank the following people for their advice and support: Ravinder Kundi, Peter Rose, Barry & Joan Cheyette, Pat & Akbar Balolia, Mark Foot, Friends and Family.

Data Sources

Carbohydrate, calorie, protein and fat values were referenced from:
- *Dietplan (version 6.60)*, Forestfield Software Limited.
- Food Standards Agency (2002) *McCance & Widdowson's: the Composition of Foods (6th Edition)*, Royal Society of Chemistry.
- Food Standards Agency *UK Food Nutrient Databank*.
- Juliette Kellow *et al* (2010) *The Calorie, Carb and Fat Bible 2010*, Weight Loss Resources Limited.

Other reference values were taken using an average of commercially available products or calculated from recipes (which are available at www.carbsandcals.com). Some values have been estimated based on similar foods. Please note that values in this book are to be used as a guide only. The authors cannot accept any liability for any consequences arising from the use of the information contained within this book. Every effort has been made to ensure figures represent a true and fair value of carbohydrate, calorie, protein and fat content of food & drinks included, but these values can vary between brands, recipes and food preparation methods.

Sustainability Policy

The authors would like to encourage people who read this book to use, where possible, Marine Stewardship Council (MSC) certified sustainable fish. The most commonly available types of fish, such as cod, have been used in this book but we would like to encourage people to use alternative, non-endangered fish such as coley or pollock. For further details please see the MSC website (www.msc.org). We would also like to encourage people to use higher welfare and free-range animal products where possible.